Chronic Disorders

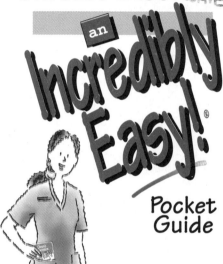

an Incredibly Easy!®

Pocket Guide

Chronic Disorders

an Incredibly Easy!®

Pocket Guide

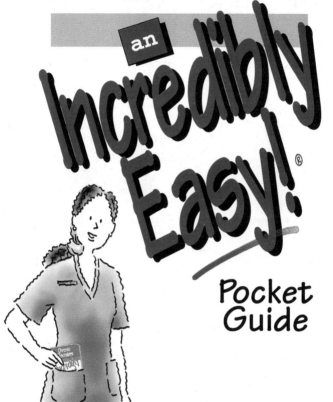

Wolters Kluwer Health | Lippincott Williams & Wilkins

Philadelphia · Baltimore · New York · London
Buenos Aires · Hong Kong · Sydney · Tokyo

Staff

Executive Publisher
Judith A. Schilling McCann, RN, MSN

Editorial Director
David Moreau

Clinical Director
Joan M. Robinson, RN, MSN

Art Director
Mary Ludwicki

Clinical Project Manager
Janet Rader Clark, RN, BSN

Editors
Diane Labus, Elizabeth Rosto

Designer
Georg W. Purvis IV

Illustrator
Bot Roda

Digital Composition Services
Diane Paluba (manager), Joyce Rossi Biletz,
Donna Morris

Associate Manufacturing Manager
Beth J. Welsh

Editorial Assistants
Karen J. Kirk, Jeri O'Shea, Linda K. Ruhf

Design Assistant
Kate Zulak

Indexer
Moose McGraw

Library of Congress Cataloging-in-Publication Data
Chronic disorders : an incredibly easy pocket guide.
        p. ; cm.
        Includes bibliographical references and index.
        1. Chronic diseases — Handbooks, manuals, etc. I. Lippincott Williams & Wilkins.
        [DNLM: 1. Chronic Disease — Handbooks.
        2. Chronic Disease — Nurses'
        Instruction. WT 39 C557 2009]
RC108.C457 2009
616'.044 — dc22
ISBN-13: 978-0-7817-8688-1 (alk. paper)
ISBN-10: 0-7817-8688-6 (alk. paper)   2008000013

Contents

Contributors and consultants

Cheryl L. Brady, RN, MSN
Assistant Professor of Nursing
Kent State University
Salem, Ohio

Kim Clevenger, MSN, RN, C
Assistant Professor of Nursing
Morehead State University
Morehead, Ky.

Kim Cooper, RN, MSN
Nursing Department Chair
Ivy Tech Community College
Terre Haute, Ind.

Shelba Durston, RN, MSN, CCRN
Nursing Instructor
San Joaquin Delta College
Stockton, Calif.

Cheryl Laskowski, DNS, APRN-BC
Assistant Professor
University of Vermont
Burlington, Vt.

Virginia Lester, RN, MSN
Assistant Professor
Angelo State University
San Angelo, Tex.

Grace G. Lewis, MS, RN, BC
Assistant Professor
Georgia Baptist College of Nursing
Mercer University
Atlanta

Kay Luft, MN, PHD-C, CCRN
Assistant Professor
Saint Luke's College
Kansas City

Phyllis M. Magaletto, MSN, APRN, BC
Instructor of Med/Surg Nursing
Cochran School of Nursing
Yonkers, N.Y.

Ann S. McQueen, MSN, CRNP
Family Nurse Practitioner
Health Link Medical Center
Southampton, Pa.

Catherine Pence, RN, MSN, CCRN
Assistant Professor
Northern Kentucky University
Highland Heights, Ky.

Noel C. Piano, RN, MS
Instructor/Coordinator
Lafayette School of Practical Nursing
Williamsburg, Va.
Adjunct Faculty
Thomas Nelson Community College
Hampton, Va.

Monica Narvaez Ramirez, MSN, RN
Nursing Instructor
University of the Incarnate Word
  School of Nursing
San Antonio, Tex.

Dana Reeves, MSN, RN
Assistant Professor
University of Arkansas
Fort Smith, Ark.

Elizabeth Richards, MSN, RN
Clinical Assistant Professor
Purdue University School of Nursing
West Lafayette, Ind.

Angela Starkweather, PHD, ACNP, CCRN, CNRN
Assistant Professor
Washington State University
  Intercollegiate College of Nursing
Spokane, Wash.

Robin R. Wilkerson, RN, PhD
Professor and Assistant Dean for
  Undergraduate Studies
University of Mississippi
School of Nursing
Jackson, Miss.

Dawn M. Zwick, MSN, CRNP
Lecturer
Kent State University
Kent, Ohio
Nurse Practitioner
Cleveland Clinic Foundation

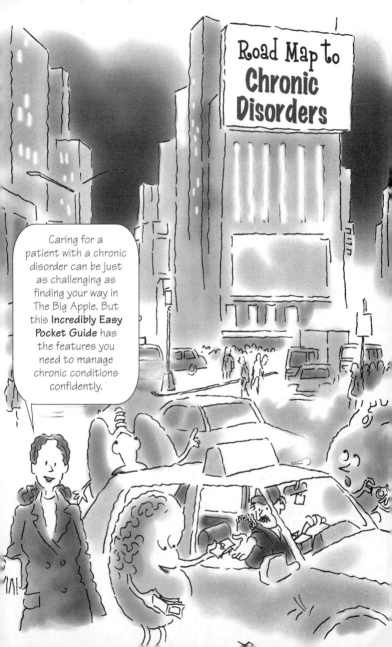

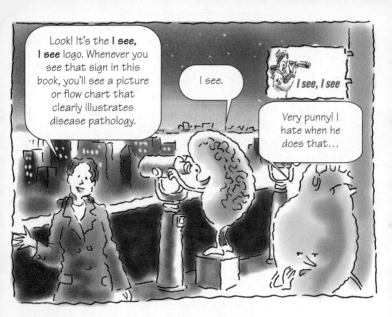
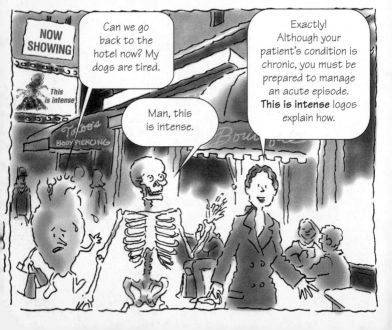

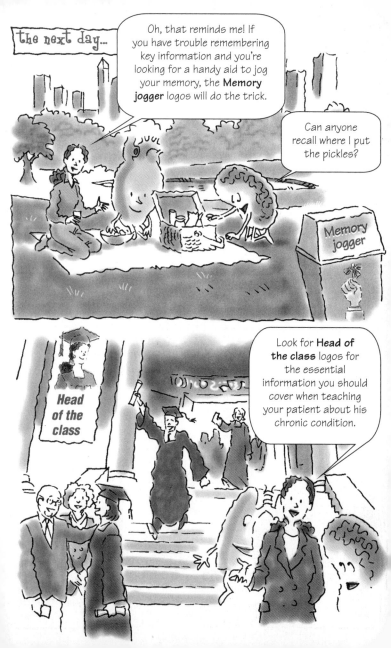

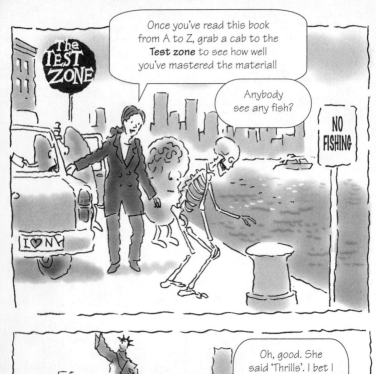
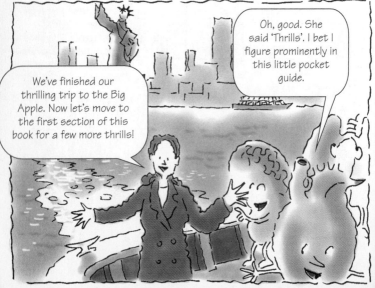

A–B

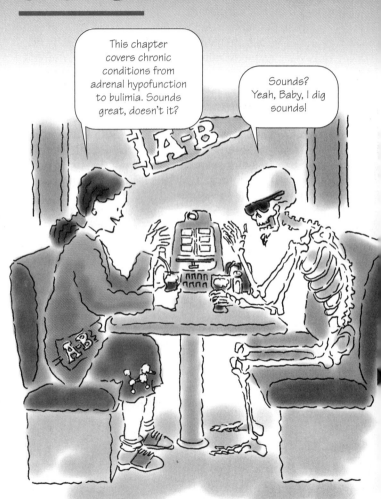

Adrenal hypofunction

- Can be primary or secondary
  - Primary hypofunction or insufficiency (Addison's disease): originates within the adrenal gland; characterized by decreased secretion of mineralocorticoids, glucocorticoids, and androgens and by complete or partial destruction of the adrenal cortex
  - Secondary hypofunction: caused by a disorder outside the adrenal gland (impaired pituitary secretion of corticotropin); characterized by decreased glucocorticoid secretion, although aldosterone secretion is unaffected
- Can lead to adrenal crisis (addisonian crisis)
  - Involves critical deficiency of mineralocorticoids and glucocorticoids
  - Generally occurs after stress, sepsis, trauma, surgery, or omission of steroid therapy in patients with chronic adrenal insufficiency

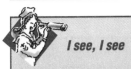

I see, I see

Understanding acute adrenal crisis

Acute adrenal crisis, the most serious complication of Addison's disease, is a life-threatening event that requires prompt assessment and immediate treatment. This flowchart highlights the underlying mechanisms responsible for this disorder.

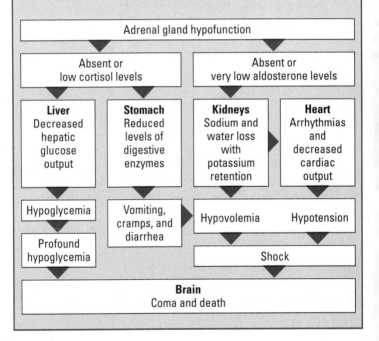

What causes it

Primary adrenal hypofunction
• Autoimmune process

- Idiopathic atrophy of adrenal glands
- Bilateral adrenalectomy
- Neoplasms, tuberculosis, or other infections (histoplasmosis, cytomegalovirus, acquired immunodeficiency syndrome)

Secondary adrenal hypofunction

- Hypopituitarism
- Abrupt withdrawal of long-term corticosteroid therapy
- Removal of corticotropin-secreting tumor

What to look for

Primary adrenal hypofunction

- Weakness and fatigue
- Weight loss and various GI disturbances, such as nausea, vomiting, anorexia, and chronic diarrhea
- Conspicuous bronze skin coloration, especially in the creases of the hands and over the metacarpophalageal, elbow, and knee joints
- Darkening of scars, areas of vitiligo (absent pigment) and increased pigmentation of the mucous membranes
- Orthostatic hypotension, decreased cardiac size and output, and a weak, irregular pulse
- Decreased stress tolerance, poor coordination, fasting hypoglycemia, and salt craving

Secondary adrenal hypofunction

- Similar effects but without hyperpigmentation and possibly no hypotension and electrolyte abnormalities

This is intense

Managing adrenal crisis

In the patient with adrenal crisis, be alert for profound weakness, fatigue, nausea, vomiting, hypotension, dehydration, and, occasionally, high fever followed by hypothermia. If you detect these signs and symptoms, follow the guidelines listed below to prevent vascular collapse, renal shutdown, coma, and, possibly, death.

• Monitor the patient's vital signs carefully, especially for hypotension, volume depletion, and other signs of shock (decreased level of consciousness and urine output).

• Promptly administer an I.V. bolus of hydrocortisone. Later doses are given I.M. or are diluted and given I.V. until the patient's condition stabilizes.

• Monitor the patient for hyperkalemia before treatment and for hypokalemia after treatment (from excessive mineralocorticoid effect).

• Monitor the patient for cardiac arrhythmias, which may be caused by a serum potassium disturbance.

• Administer vasopressors (if necessary) to treat hypotension unresponsive to initial treatment.

• If the patient also has diabetes, check blood glucose levels periodically, because steroid replacement may require insulin dosage adjustments.

• Document the patient's weight and intake and output carefully because he may have volume depletion. Until the onset of mineralocorticoid effect, force fluids to replace excessive fluid loss.

• After the crisis, administer maintenance doses of hydrocortisone, as ordered, to preserve physiologic stability.

How it's treated

• Lifelong cortisone or hydrocortisone administration for corticosteroid replacement in primary or secondary adrenal hypofunction

- Oral fludrocortisone, a synthetic mineralocorticoid, to prevent dangerous dehydration, hypotension, hyponatremia, and hyperkalemia (Addison's disease)

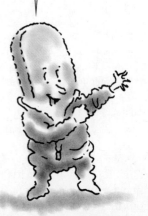

Alcohol dependence

- The need for daily intake of alcohol for day-to-day functioning or a regular pattern of heavy drinking that's limited to weekends, with periods of sobriety during the week
- Associated with impaired social and occupational functioning

What causes it

- Biologic factors: genetic or biochemical abnormalities; nutritional deficiencies; endocrine imbalances; and allergic responses
- Psychological factors: urge to drink to reduce anxiety or symptoms of mental illness; desire to avoid responsibility in familial, social, and work relationships; and need to bolster self-esteem
- Sociocultural factors: availability of alcohol; group or peer pressure; excessively stressful lifestyle; and social attitudes that approve of frequent excessive drinking

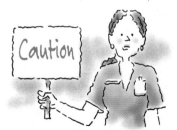

Regular patterns of heavy drinking indicate a problem. Dependence on alcohol can have biological, psychological, or sociocultural causes.

Caution

Complications of alcohol use

Alcohol can damage body tissues by its direct irritating effects, by changes that take place in the body during its metabolism, by aggravation of existing disease, by accidents occurring during intoxication, and by interactions between the substance and drugs. Such tissue damage can cause the complications outlined below.

Cardiopulmonary
- Cardiac arrhythmias
- Cardiomyopathy
- Chronic obstructive pulmonary disease
- Essential hypertension
- Pneumonia

Hematologic
- Anemia
- Leukopenia
- Reduced number of phagocytes

Hepatic
- Alcoholic hepatitis
- Cirrhosis
- Fatty liver

GI
- Chronic diarrhea
- Esophageal cancer
- Esophageal varices
- Esophagitis
- Gastric ulcers
- Gastritis
- GI bleeding
- Malabsorption
- Pancreatitis

Neurologic
- Alcoholic dementia
- Alcoholic hallucinosis
- Alcohol withdrawal delirium
- Korsakoff's syndrome
- Peripheral neuropathy
- Seizure disorders
- Subdural hematoma
- Wernicke's encephalopathy

Psychiatric
- Abuse of multiple substances
- Amotivational syndrome
- Depression
- Impaired social and occupational functioning
- Suicide

Other
- Beriberi
- Fetal alcohol syndrome
- Hypoglycemia
- Increased incidence of pulmonary infections
- Infertility
- Leg and foot ulcers
- Myopathies
- Prostatitis
- Sexual performance difficulties

What to look for

- History of daily or episodic alcohol use with inability to discontinue or reduce intake
- Episodes of anesthesia or amnesia (blackouts) and episodes of violence during intoxication, as well as impaired social and familial relationships and impaired occupational performance
- Symptoms of malaise, dyspepsia, mood swings, or depression
- Increased incidence of infection
- Poor hygiene and untreated or frequent injuries (such as cigarette burns, fractures, and bruises) that the patient can't fully explain
- Secretive or manipulative behavior and denial, hostility, or rationalization when confronted
- Signs and symptoms of withdrawal beginning shortly after abstinence or reduction of alcohol intake and lasting for 5 to 7 days

How it's treated

- Total abstinence from alcohol (the only effective treatment)
- Supportive programs that offer detoxification, rehabilitation, and aftercare, including continued involvement in Alcoholics Anonymous
- Prevention of pleasurable effects of increased endorphins produced by alcohol intake through the use of naltrexone, an opiate antagonist
- Aversion or deterrent therapy using disulfiram, which produces immediate and potentially fatal distress if the patient consumes alcohol up to 2 weeks after taking it
- B-complex vitamins to correct nutritional deficiencies

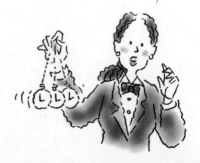

Alzheimer's disease

- Degenerative disorder of cerebral cortex (especially frontal lobe and hippocampus) that's considered primary progressive form of dementia
- Accounts for more than half of all cases of dementia
- Has poor prognosis

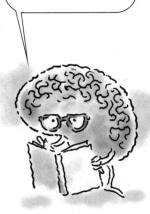

It says here that Alzheimer's disease accounts for more than half of all dementia cases.

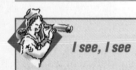

I see, I see

Abnormal cell structures in Alzheimer's disease

How and why neurons die in Alzheimer's disease is largely unknown. The brain tissue of patients with Alzheimer's disease exhibits these three distinct, characteristic features.

Granulovacuolar degeneration
Granulovacuolar degeneration occurs inside the neurons of the hippocampus. An abnormally high number of fluid-filled spaces (vacuoles) enlarges the cell's body, possibly causing the cell to die.

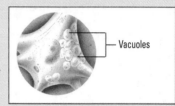

Neurofibrillary tangles
Neurofibrillary tangles are bundles of filaments inside the neuron that abnormally twist around one another. They're found in the brain areas associated with memory and learning (hippocampus), fear and aggression (amygdala), and thinking (cerebral cortex). These tangles may play a role in the memory loss and personality changes that commonly occur in Alzheimer's disease.

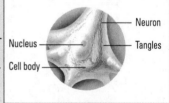

Amyloid plaques
Also called *senile plaques,* amyloid plaques are found outside neurons in the extracellular space of the cerebral cortex and hippocampus. They contain a core of beta amyloid protein surrounded by abnormal nerve endings (neurites).

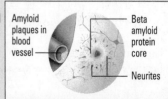

What causes it

- Exact cause unknown
- Possible neurochemical factors, including deficiencies in the neurotransmitters acetylcholine, serotonin, somatostatin, and norepinephrine
- Environmental factors, including repeated head trauma and exposure to aluminum or manganese
- Genetic factors

What to look for

Initial stage

- Gradual loss of recent and remote memory
- Disorientation (time, date, and place)
- Flattening of affect and personality

Progressive stages

- Impaired cognition
- Inability to concentrate
- Difficulty with abstraction and judgment
- Inability to perform activities of daily living
- Restlessness and agitation
- Personality changes
- Nocturnal awakening and wandering
- Severe deterioration in memory, language, and motor function
- Loss of coordination
- Inability to write or speak
- Loss of eye contact
- Acute confusion, agitation, compulsive behavior or fearfulness
- Emotional lability
- Urinary and fecal incontinence

How it's treated

- Cholinesterase inhibition therapy to help improve memory deficits
- N-methyl-D-aspartate receptor antagonist therapy to improve memory and learning of patients with moderate to severe Alzheimer's disease
- Antidepressants to improve mood and reduce irritability
- Antipsychotics to treat hallucinations, delusions, aggression, hostility, and uncooperativeness
- Antioxidant therapy (vitamin E therapy under current study) to delay disease effects
- Anxiolytics to treat anxiety, restlessness, verbally disruptive behavior, and resistance
- Behavioral interventions (simplifying environment, tasks, and routines) to prevent agitation
- Effective communication strategies to ensure continued communication between patient and family
- Teaching aids, safety needs, and social service and community resources to educate caregivers and provide legal and financial advice and support

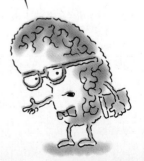

Alzheimer's disease is linked to environmental and genetic factors that cause progressive dementia.

Amyotrophic lateral sclerosis

- Chronic, progressively debilitating disease, commonly called Lou Gehrig disease
- Most common form of motor neuron disease causing muscular atrophy
- Onset usually between ages 40 and 60
- Twice as common in men as in women

I see, I see

Understanding ALS

ALS progressively destroys upper and lower motor neurons (including anterior horn cells of the spinal cord, upper motor neurons of the cerebral cortex, and motor nuclei of the brain stem).

ALS may begin when glutamate (primary excitatory neurotransmitter of central nervous system) accumulates to toxic levels at synapses.

Affected motor units are no longer innervated; progressive degeneration of axons causes loss of myelin.

Nonfunctional scar tissue replaces normal neuronal tissue; denervation leads to muscle fiber atrophy and motor neuron degeneration.

What causes it

- Exact cause unknown; 5% to 10% of cases have genetic component
- Possible contributing mechanisms:
  - slow-acting virus
  - nutritional deficiency related to disturbance in enzyme metabolism
  - unknown mechanism that causes buildup of excess glutamine in CSF
  - autoimmune disorder

What to look for

- Progressive loss of muscle strength and coordination
- Eventual inability to perform activities of daily living
- Fasciculations, muscle atrophy and weakness, especially in the feet and hands
- Impaired speech
- Difficulty chewing, swallowing, and breathing
- Choking and excessive drooling
- Depression in reaction to the disease

How it's treated

- Supportive medical intervention (ALS has no cure):
  - diazepam, dantrolene, or baclofen to decrease spasticity
  - thyrotropin-releasing hormone to temporarily improve motor function
  - riluzole to modulate glutamate activity and slow disease progression
- Respiratory, speech, and physical therapy and assistive devices to maintain as much function as possible
- Psychological support to assist with coping
- Rehabilitation program to maintain independence as long as possible
- Gastrostomy to facilitate nutritional support in patients at risk for aspiration

- Mechanical ventilation for respiratory support, if the patient wishes
- Referral to hospice or local ALS support group as supportive care for patient and family (to manage care as the disease progresses and to assist with decisions about artificial ventilation and life-sustaining treatments)

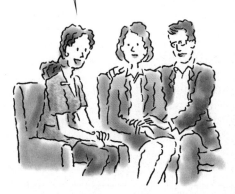

Patients with ALS and their families can benefit greatly from joining support groups.

Anemia, iron deficiency

- Oxygen-transport disorder characterized by deficiency in hemoglobin synthesis
- Most common in premenopausal women, infants, children, and adolescents (especially girls)

I see, I see

Understanding iron deficiency anemia

Iron deficiency anemia occurs when the supply of iron is inadequate for optimal RBC formation, resulting in smaller (microcytic) cells with less color (hypochromic) on staining and, in severe disease, elongated, cigar-shaped cells. Body stores of iron become depleted, and the concentration of serum transferrin (which binds with and transports iron) decreases. Insufficient iron stores lead to a depleted RBC mass with subnormal hemoglobin concentration and, in turn, subnormal oxygen-carrying capacity of the blood.

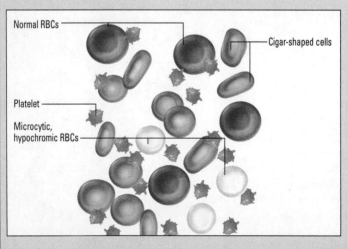

What causes it
- Inadequate dietary intake of iron (less than 2 mg/day)

Risk factors
- Prolonged, unsupplemented (iron) breast- or bottle-feeding or during rapid growth phases
- Iron malabsorption from chronic diarrhea, partial or total gastrectomy; or malabsorption syndromes such as celiac disease
- Blood loss from drug-induced GI bleeding, heavy menses, traumatic hemorrhage, peptic ulcer, cancer, excessive blood sampling, sequestration, varices
- Pregnancy (diverts maternal iron to fetus for erythropoiesis)
- Intravascular hemolysis-induced hemoglobinuria, paroxysmal nocturnal hemoglobinuria
- Mechanical trauma to RBCs from prosthetic heart valve or vena cava filters

What to look for
- Decreased oxygen-carrying capacity of blood due to decreased hemoglobin levels
  - Dyspnea on exertion
  - Fatigue and listlessness
  - Pallor
  - Inability to concentrate
  - Irritability
  - Headache
  - Susceptibility to infection
- Increased cardiac output and tachycardia from decreased perfusion
- Nails that are coarsely ridged, spoon-shaped, brittle, due to decreased capillary circulation
- Sore, red, burning tongue
- Sore, dry skin at corners of mouth

How it's treated

- Identification of underlying cause to permit appropriate treatment of the anemia
- Iron replacement therapy, which may include oral iron preparation (treatment of choice) or combined iron and ascorbic acid (enhances iron absorption) to ensure adequate intake of iron
- Administration of parenteral iron for those having problems with oral medication (noncompliance, need for more iron than can be given orally, malabsorption); also given to achieve maximum rate of hemoglobin regeneration
- Careful medication monitoring to ensure compliance with prescribed therapy
- Administration of oral supplements at mealtimes to decrease gastric irritation

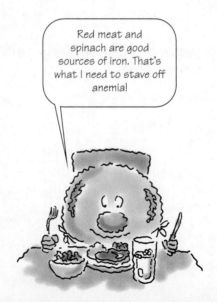

Anemia, pernicious

- Most common type of megaloblastic anemia
- Characterized by lack of intrinsic factor (needed to absorb vitamin B_{12}) and widespread RBC destruction
- Characteristic manifestations that subside with treatment; possible permanent neurologic deficits

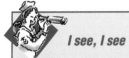

I see, I see

Understanding pernicious anemia

Pernicious anemia is characterized by decreased production of hydrochloric acid in the stomach and a deficiency of intrinsic factor, which is normally secreted by the parietal cells of the gastric mucosa and is essential for vitamin B_{12} absorption in the ileum. The resulting vitamin B_{12} deficiency inhibits cell growth, particularly of RBCs, leading to production of few, deformed RBCs with poor oxygen-carrying capacity. RBCs are abnormally large due to excess ribonucleic acid production of the hemoglobin. Pernicious anemia also causes neurologic damage by impairing myelin formation.

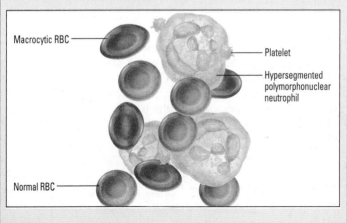

Macrocytic RBC

Platelet

Hypersegmented polymorphonuclear neutrophil

Normal RBC

What causes it

- Deficiency of vitamin B_{12}

Risk factors

- Genetic predisposition
- Immunologically related diseases (thyroiditis, myxedema, Graves' disease)
- Partial gastrectomy
- Aging (progressive loss of vitamin B_{12} absorption, usually beginning after age 50)

What to look for

- Initially insidious onset
- Classic triad of symptoms:
  - Weakness
  - Sore tongue
  - Numbness and tingling in the extremities
- Pale oral mucous membranes
- Faintly jaundiced sclera and skin
- Increased susceptibility to infection
- Interference of nerve impulse transmission from vitamin B_{12} deficiency
  - Lack of coordination, ataxia, impaired fine finger movement
  - Altered vision, taste, and hearing; optic muscle atrophy
  - Loss of bowel and bladder control; impotence (males)
- Nausea, vomiting, anorexia, weight loss, flatulence, diarrhea and constipation from gastric mucosal atrophy and decreased hydrochloric acid production
- Palpations, wide pulse pressure, dyspnea, tachycardia, premature beats, and, eventually, heart failure

How it's treated

- Vitamin B_{12} replacement (lifelong) to ensure adequate intake

- Concomitant iron and folic acid replacement to prevent iron deficiency anemia
- Bed rest for extreme fatigue until hemoglobin level rises
- Blood transfusions for dangerously low hemoglobin level
- Digoxin, diuretics, low-sodium diet to treat heart failure if it occurs
- Antibiotics to combat infection
- Educational materials to promote compliance

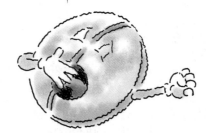

I think I'll hop back into bed for a few days until my hemoglobin level starts to rise.

Ankylosing spondylitis

- Progressive inflammatory disease that primarily affects the sacroiliac, apophyseal, and costovertebral joints and adjacent soft tissue
- Deterioration of bone and cartilage that can lead to fusion of the spine or peripheral joints
- Unpredictable progression, with periods of remission, exacerbation, or arrest at any stage

What causes it
- No clear cause (evidence suggests familial and immunologic components)

What to look for
- Initially intermittent lower back pain, usually most severe in the morning or after inactivity
- Hip and spine deformity and associated limited range of motion (ROM)
- Tenderness over the inflammation site and peripheral arthritis
- Mild fatigue
- Fever
- Anorexia or weight loss
- Aortic insufficiency and cardiomegaly
- Upper lobe pulmonary fibrosis and dyspnea
- Pain and limited chest expansion due to involvement of the costovertebral joints
- Presence of HLA-B27 human leukocyte antigen; negative rheumatoid factor; and elevated sedimentation rate, alkaline phosphatase, and serum immunoglobulin A

How it's treated
- Anti-inflammatory analgesics, corticosteroid therapy, and tumor necrosis factor inhibitors for symptom control

- Cytotoxic drugs that block cell growth for patients who don't respond well to or who are dependent on high doses of corticosteroids
- Surgical hip replacement or spinal wedge osteotomy in severe cases
- Physical and occupational therapy to help maintain function and minimize deformity
- Assistive devices to aid independence

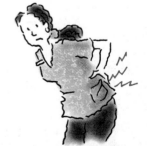

Anorexia nervosa

- Self-imposed starvation, resulting from a distorted body image and an intense, irrational fear of gaining weight
- Preoccupation with body size and expressions of dissatisfaction with a particular physical appearance aspect
- Rarely, true loss of appetite
- Two types
  - Restriction of eating that includes refusal to eat, compulsive exercising, self-induced vomiting, or abuse of laxatives or diuretics
  - Binging and purging

What causes it

- No identified cause (genetic, social, and psychological factors have been implicated)
- Association with other psychiatric disorders, such as obsessive-compulsive disorder, depression, and anxiety

What to look for

- Weight loss of 25% or more with no organic reason combined with a morbid dread of being fat and a compulsion to be thin
- Tendency to be angry and ritualistic
- May have obsession with food, preparing elaborate meals for others
- Social regression, fear of failure, depression
- Amenorrhea, infertility, sleep alterations, intolerance to cold

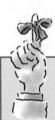

Memory jogger

The word HUNGER is your guidepost to the major features of anorexia nervosa.

H Has an obsession with food and weight

U Underweight or emaciated

N Needs go unmet because of controlling parents or family conflict

G Gross distortion of body image

E Exercises, vomits, or uses laxatives and diuretics to lose weight

R Refuses to eat

- Hypotension and bradycardia
- Emaciated appearance, with skeletal muscle atrophy, loss of fatty tissue, atrophy of breast tissue, blotchy or sallow skin, lanugo on the face and body, and dryness of scalp hair
- Calluses on the knuckles, and abrasions and scars on the dorsum of the hand from tooth injury during self-induced vomiting if the patient is also bulimic
- Bowel distention and constipation
- Multiple laboratory abnomalities and ECG changes

How it's treated

- Behavior modification to encourage weight gain
- Restricted activity, with gradual increase with weight gain and medical stability
- Nutritional support, including vitamin and mineral supplements, a reasonable diet with supplements, parenteral hyperalimentation if necessary
- Group, family, or individual therapy to address underlying problems

Anxiety disorder, generalized

- Anxiety: a feeling of apprehension, dread, or uneasiness in reaction to an internal threat
- Generalized anxiety disorder: uncontrollable, unreasonable worry that persists for at least 6 months and narrows perceptions or interferes with normal functioning

What causes it

- No identified cause (possibly, a combination of genetic, biochemical, neuroanatomic, and psychological factors plus life experiences)

What to look for

- Varying signs and symptoms, depending on the disorder's severity
  - Unusual self-awareness and alertness to the environment (mild anxiety)
  - Selective inattention, with the ability to concentrate on a single task (moderate anxiety)
  - Inability to concentrate on more than a part of a task (severe anxiety)
  - Complete loss of concentration and unintelligible speech (panic state)
- Trembling, muscle aches and spasms, headaches, and inability to relax
- Shortness of breath, tachycardia, sweating, and abdominal complaints
- Eating and sleeping difficulties

How it's treated

- Medications: benzodiazepines, buspirone, selective serotonin reuptake inhibitors
- Psychotherapy
- Relaxation techniques

Aortic insufficiency

- Incomplete closure of aortic valve
- Usually caused by scarring or retraction of valve leaflets

I see, I see

Understanding aortic insufficiency

In aortic insufficiency, blood flows back into the left ventricle during diastole, causing fluid overload in the ventricle, which dilates and hypertrophies. The excess volume causes fluid overload in the left atrium and, lastly, the pulmonary system. Left-sided heart failure and pulmonary edema eventually result.

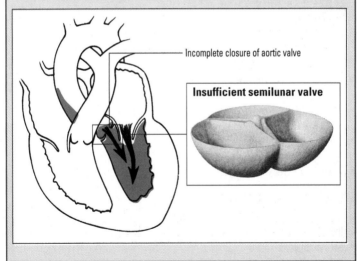

Incomplete closure of aortic valve

Insufficient semilunar valve

What causes it
- Rheumatic fever
- Marfan syndrome
- Ankylosing spondylitis
- Syphilis
- Ventricular septal defect

What to look for
- Increased pulmonary venous pressure and cardiac dysfunction
  - Exertional dyspnea
  - Orthopnea
  - Paroxysmal nocturnal dyspnea
- Left ventricular dysfunction
  - Fatigue
  - Exercise intolerance
  - Cough
  - Left-sided heart failure
  - "Pulsating" nail beds (Quincke's sign)
  - S_3 heart sound
- Inadequate coronary perfusion
  - Angina
- Hyperdynamic and tachycardic left ventricle
  - Palpitations
- Low diastolic pressure
  - Widened pulse pressure
- Diastolic blowing murmur at left sternal border

How it's treated
- Vasodilators to reduce systolic load and regurgitant volume
- Digoxin, low-sodium diet, and diuretics to treat left-sided heart failure
- Prophylactic antibiotics before and after surgery or dental care to prevent endocarditis
- Nitroglycerin to relieve angina

- Valve replacement of diseased aortic valve
- Anticoagulation to prevent thrombus formation on diseased or prosthetic valve

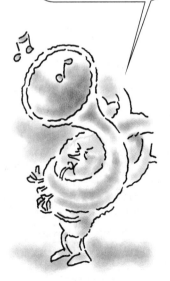

Listen for a diastolic blowing murmur at the left sternal border in a patient with aortic insufficiency.

Aortic stenosis

- Narrowing of aortic valve
- Classified as acquired or rheumatic
- Classic triad of angina pectoris, syncope, and dyspnea

I see, I see

Understanding aortic stenosis

Stenosis of the aortic valve results in impedance to forward blood flow. The left ventricle requires greater pressure to open the aortic valve. The added workload increases the demand for oxygen, and diminished cardiac output causes poor coronary artery perfusion, ischemia of the left ventricle, left ventricular hypertrophy, and left-sided heart failure.

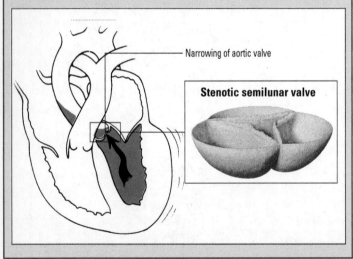

Narrowing of aortic valve

Stenotic semilunar valve

What causes it

- Idiopathic fibrosis and calcification
- Congenital aortic bicuspid valve
- Rheumatic fever
- Atherosclerosis

What to look for

- Exertional dyspnea due to abnormal diastolic function
- Angina secondary to increased oxygen requirement by hypertrophic myocardium and diminished oxygen delivery secondary to compression of coronary vessels
- Syncope related to systemic vasodilation or arrhythmias
- Left-sided heart failure
- Harsh, rasping, crescendo-decrescendo systolic murmur

How it's treated

- Periodic, noninvasive evaluation to monitor valve narrowing
- Digoxin to control atrial fibrillation
- Low-sodium diet and diuretics to treat left-sided heart failure
- Prophylactic antibiotics before and after surgery or dental care to prevent endocarditis
- Percutaneous balloon aortic valvuloplasty to reduce stenosis
- Aortic valve replacement to replace diseased valve
- Anticoagulation to protect against thrombus formation on diseased or prosthetic valve

Arterial occlusive disease

- Obstruction or narrowing of the lumen of the aorta and its major branches, which interrupts blood flow, usually to the legs and feet
- Prognosis: depends on location of the occlusion and development of collateral circulation

What causes it

- Complication of atherosclerosis
- May be endogenous (due to emboli formation or thrombosis) or exogenous (due to trauma or fracture)
- Predisposing factors: smoking, age, hypertension, hyperlipidemia, diabetes, and family history of cardiovascular disorders

What to look for

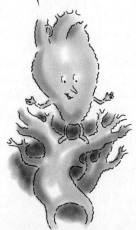

Blood needs to be able to flow freely for me to do my best work!

- Signs and symptoms depend on the site of the occlusion
- Sensory and motor deficits; transient ischemic attacks
- Signs of ischemia (pain and cold, pale limb, decreased or absent peripheral pulses) and gangrene
- Auscultatory bruit over the affected vessel
- Intermittent claudication
- Impotence
- In mesenteric artery occlusion: diarrhea, leukocytosis, nausea and vomiting, abdominal pain, shock
- Impaired nail and hair growth
- Skin ulceration

How it's treated

- Supportive measures, such as smoking cessation, hypertension control, and mild exercise
- Antiplatelet therapy with ticlopidine or clopidogrel and aspirin
- Pentoxifylline and cilostazol for intermittent claudication
- Surgery to restore circulation to the affected area
- Amputation if surgery fails or if gangrene, persistent infection, or intractable pain develops
- Bowel resection of necrotic area after blood flow restoration to mesenteric artery

This is intense

Managing an acute arterial occlusion

Although arterial occlusion is usually chronic, an acute exacerbation can develop, most commonly due to a clot. When caring for a patient with an acute arterial occlusion, follow these guidelines:
- Place the affected limb flat or below the level of the heart.
- Administer thrombolytic or heparin therapy, as ordered.
- Prepare the patient for possible surgery to restore circulation to the affected area.

Preoperative interventions
- Assess the patient's circulatory status by checking for the most distal pulses and by inspecting his skin color and temperature.
- Provide pain relief as needed.
- Administer I.V. heparin.
- Wrap the patient's affected limb in soft cotton batting, and reposition it frequently to prevent pressure on any one area.
- Strictly avoid elevation or applying heat to the affected area.
- Watch for signs of fluid and electrolyte imbalance, and monitor intake and output for signs of renal failure (urine output less than 30 ml/hr).

(continued)

Managing an acute arterial occlusion *(continued)*

• If the patient has carotid, innominate, vertebral, or subclavian artery occlusion, monitor for signs of stroke, such as numbness in his arm or leg and intermittent blindness.

Postoperative interventions

• Monitor the patient's vital signs. Continuously assess his circulatory status. Watch closely for signs of hemorrhage (tachycardia and hypotension), and check dressings for excessive bleeding.

• Assess the patient's neurologic status frequently for changes in level of consciousness, muscle strength, and pupil size.

• Monitor the patient's intake and output (low urine output may indicate damage to renal arteries during surgery).

• Watch for signs of mesenteric artery occlusion (severe abdominal pain) as well as cardiac arrhythmias, which may precipitate embolus formation.

• After amputation, check the patient's stump carefully for drainage and record its color and amount and the time. Elevate the stump, as ordered, and administer adequate pain medication. Because phantom limb pain is common, explain this phenomenon to the patient.

Asbestosis

- Diffuse interstitial pulmonary fibrosis secondary to asbestos fiber inhalation
- May develop 15 to 20 years after regular exposure has ended
- A potent cocarcinogen that significantly increases a smoker's risk of lung cancer

What causes it

- Prolonged exposure to airborne particles, which causes pleural plaques and tumors of the pleura and peritoneum
- Swelling of airways and development of fibrosis from foreign material, inflammation, and chronic irritation

Risk factors

- History of occupation in mining, milling, construction, fireproofing, or textile industry (typically for more than 10 years)
- Exposure to paints, plastics, or brake and clutch linings
- For family members: exposure to fibrous dust from clothing of asbestos workers

What to look for

- Dyspnea on exertion, pleuritic chest pain, recurrent respiratory infections, basilar crackles and tachypnea
- Cough (productive in smokers)
- Clubbed fingers
- Abnormal chest X-ray and pulmonary function studies

How it's treated

- Chest physiotherapy to relieve symptoms
- Aerosol therapy to liquefy and mobilize secretions
- Increased fluid intake to thin secretions
- Antibiotics to treat respiratory tract infections
- Oxygen to relieve hypoxia
- Diuretics to decrease edema, if needed

- Digoxin to enhance cardiac output if needed
- Salt restriction to prevent fluid retention in patients with cor pulmonale

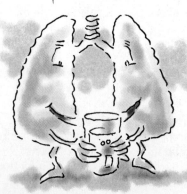

Asthma

- Chronic inflammatory airway disorder characterized by airflow obstruction and airway hyperresponsiveness to multiple stimuli
- Type of chronic obstructive pulmonary disease (COPD)
- May result from sensitivity to extrinsic or intrinsic allergens

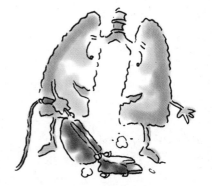

I see, I see

Understanding asthma

In asthma, hyperresponsiveness of the airways and bronchospasms occur. These illustrations show how an asthma attack progresses.

1. Histamine (H) attaches to receptor sites in larger bronchi, causing swelling of the smooth muscles.

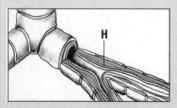

2. Leukotrienes (L) attach to receptor sites in the smaller bronchi and cause swelling of smooth muscle there. Leukotrienes also cause prostaglandins to travel through the bloodstream to the lungs, where they enhance histamine's effects.

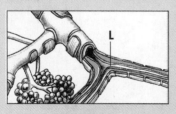

3. Histamine stimulates the mucous membranes to secrete excessive mucus, further narrowing the bronchial lumen. On inhalation, the narrowed bronchial lumen can still expand slightly; on exhalation, however, the increased intrathoracic pressure closes the bronchial lumen completely.

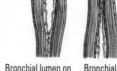

Bronchial lumen on inhalation   Bronchial lumen on exhalation

4. Mucus fills lung bases, inhibiting alveolar ventilation. Blood is shunted to alveoli in other parts of the lungs, but it still can't compensate for diminished ventilation.

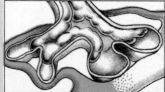

What causes it

Extrinsic allergens

- Pollen
- Animal dander
- House dust or mold
- Kapok or feather pillows
- Food additives containing sulfites
- Other sensitizing substances

Intrinsic allergens

- Irritants
- Emotional stress
- Fatigue
- Endocrine changes
- Temperature variations
- Humidity variations
- Exposure to noxious fumes
- Anxiety
- Coughing or laughing
- Genetic factors

What to look for

- Bronchial constriction
  - Sudden dyspnea
  - Wheezing
  - Tightness in chest
  - Diminished breath sounds
- Excessive mucus production
  - Coughing
  - Thick, clear or yellow sputum
- Hypoxemia
  - Rapid pulse
  - Tachypnea

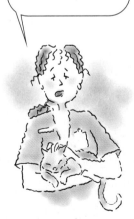

An allergy to pet dander can really set off an asthma attack!

– Use of accessory respiratory muscles

How it's treated

- Identification and avoidance of precipitating factors (environmental allergens or irritants) to prevent asthma attacks
- Desensitization to specific antigens to decrease severity of asthma attacks during future exposure to allergen
- Bronchodilators to decrease bronchoconstriction, reduce bronchial airway edema, and increase pulmonary ventilation
- Corticosteroids to decrease inflammation and edema of airways
- Mast cell stabilizers to block acute obstructive effects of antigen exposure (inhibit degranulation of mast cells, thereby preventing release of chemical mediators responsible for anaphylaxis)
- Leukotriene modifiers and leukotriene receptor antagonists (may be used as adjunctive therapy to avoid high-dose inhaled corticosteroids or when patient is noncompliant with corticosteroid therapy) to inhibit potent bronchoconstriction and inflammatory effects of cysteinyl leukotrienes
- Anticholinergic bronchodilators to block acetylcholine (another chemical mediator)
- Relaxation exercises (yoga) to increase circulation and help the patient relax and relieve stress
- Personalized asthma action plan with instructions for daily treatment and strategies to recognize and manage exacerbations to improve self-monitoring and management

This is intense

Managing an asthma attack

If your patient is having an acute asthma attack, act quickly to decrease bronchoconstriction and airway edema and increase pulmonary ventilation. Follow these guidelines:
• Assess the severity of the attack by checking for worsening shortness of breath, tight and dry cough, wheezing, and chest tightness. Cyanosis, confusion, and lethargy indicate the onset of respiratory failure.
• Assess for tachycardia, tachypnea, and diaphoresis.
• Administer the prescribed treatments and assess the patient's response.
• Place the patient in high Fowler's position and encourage pursed-lip and diaphragmatic breathing. Help him to relax.
• Monitor the patient's vital signs.
• Administer humidified oxygen by nasal cannula; adjust oxygen according to vital signs and arterial blood gas levels.
• Anticipate endotracheal intubation and mechanical ventilation if the patient fails to maintain adequate oxygenation.
• Observe the frequency and severity of your patient's cough, and note whether it's productive.
• Auscultate his lungs, noting adventitious or absent breath sounds.
• Perform postural drainage and chest percussion, if tolerated.
• Suction as needed.
• Treat dehydration with I.V. fluids until the patient can tolerate oral fluids, to loosen secretions.
  If status asthmaticus develops:
• Monitor the patient closely for respiratory failure.
• Administer oxygen, bronchodilators, epinephrine, corticosteroids, and nebulizer therapies as ordered.
• Expect intubation and mechanical ventilation if the partial pressure of arterial carbon dioxide increases or respiratory failure occurs.

Atrial fibrillation

- Chaotic, asynchronous electrical activity in the atrial tissue due to the firing of multiple impulses from numerous ectopic pacemakers
- Absence of P waves on electrocardiogram
- Irregularly irregular ventricular response

Recognizing atrial fibrillation

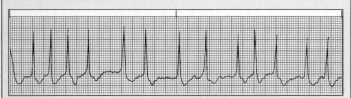

Rhythm
- Atrial: Irregularly irregular
- Ventricular: Irregularly irregular

Rate
- Atrial: Almost indiscernible, usually above 400 beats/minute, and far exceeding ventricular rate because most impulses aren't conducted through the atrioventricular junction
- Ventricular: Usually 100 to 150 beats/minute but can be below 100 beats/minute

P wave
- Absent
- Replaced by baseline fibrillatory waves that represent atrial tetanization from rapid atrial depolarizations

PR interval
- Indiscernible

QRS complex
- Duration and configuration usually normal

T wave
- Indiscernible

QT interval
- Not measurable

Other
- Atrial rhythm may vary between fibrillatory line and flutter waves, called *atrial fib-flutter.*
- May be difficult to differentiate atrial fibrillation from multifocal atrial tachycardia.

What causes it

- Acute MI
- Atrial septal defect
- Cardiomyopathy
- Coronary artery disease
- Hypertension
- Pericarditis
- Valvular heart disease (especially mitral valve disease)
- Rheumatic heart disease
- Cardiac surgery
- COPD
- Drugs such as aminophylline
- Digoxin toxicity
- Endogenous catecholamine release during exercise
- Hyperthyroidism

Triggers

- Alcohol
- Caffeine
- Nicotine

What to look for

- Radial pulse slower than apical pulse
- Irregularly irregular pulse rhythm
- Abnormal ECG
- Hypotension, light-headedness, and heart failure with rapid rate and decreased cardiac output
- Pulmonary, cerebral, or other thromboembolic event
- Possibly no symptoms of chronic atrial fibrillation in a patient able to compensate for decreased cardiac output

How it's treated

- Synchronized electrical cardioversion if the patient is hemodynamically unstable
  - Should be performed immediately (most successful within first 48 hours of onset)

- – Should not be perfomed after 48 hours of onset unless patient has been adequately anticoagulated because of the risk of thromboembolism
- Beta-adrenergic blockers (such as metoprolol), calcium channel blockers (such as diltiazem), digoxin, or amiodarone to control ventricular rate, encourage chemical cardioversion, and maintain sinus rhythm after electrical cardioversion
- Radio-frequency ablation therapy for symptomatic atrial fibrillation that doesn't respond to treatments above
- Lifelong rate control and anticoagulation therapy for asymptomatic atrial fibrillation that doesn't respond to treatments above

Head of the class

Chronic anticoagulation therapy

The most common anticoagulant used for chronic therapy is warfarin. Once the physician and the patient determine that the benefits of therapy outweigh the risks, the patient and his family will need education for its safe use. In addition to face-to-face instruction, provide the patient with written materials that include the following information and instructions:

• Periodic blood tests are necessary to monitor the drug's effects.
• Take a missed dose as soon as possible and then resume your normal schedule. Take a double dose only if directed by your physician.
• Keep a written record of test results and current dosing instructions. Doses can change frequently, especially at the start of therapy.
• Report nosebleeds, excessive bleeding from the gums or cuts, easy bruising, blood in urine, black tarry stools, or coffee-ground vomitus.
• Report all prescription and over-the counter medications and dietary supplements to your physician.
• Inform all health care providers that you take an anticoagulant, especially before surgery, dental work, or tests.
• Limit alcohol use to one or two drinks.
• Wear medical identification indicating that you use a "blood thinner."
• To prevent bleeding, avoid contact sports and use caution when brushing teeth and shaving.
• Follow a balanced diet that includes green, leafy vegetables, which are rich in vitamin K.

Attention deficit hyperactivity disorder

- Difficulty focusing attention or engaging in quiet, passive activities, or both
- Present at birth but difficult to diagnose before age 4 or 5
- May have attention deficit without hyperactivity

What causes it
- Genetic tendency
- Possibly related to neurotransmitter disturbances due to reduced blood flow within the striated area of the brain

What to look for
- Hyperactivity over a long period that occurs in at least two settings, such as home and school or work
- Easy distractibility
- Impulsive, emotionally labile, explosive, or irritable behavior
- Sporadic school or work performance unrelated to intelligence
- Jump from one partly completed project, thought, or task to another

How it's treated
- Behavior modification
- Coaching
- External structure
- Use of planning and organizing systems
- Supportive psychotherapy
- Stimulants to relieve symptoms, possibly in combination with antipsychotics
- Tricyclic antidepressants, mood stabilizers, or beta-adrenergic blockers to help control symptoms

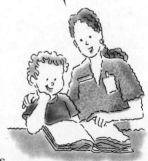

Children with ADHD have difficulty concentrating on their own.

Autism

- Developmental disorder characterized by inappropriate responses to the environment
- Pronounced impairments in language, communication, and social interaction
- Usually diagnosed by age 3
- Lasts throughout life

What causes it

- No known cause
- Possible causes: abnormalities in brain structure or function, medical problems, and genetic predisposition

What to look for

- Reports from parents that their infant doesn't appear to hear
- Normal development until about age 2, then rapid regression
- Impaired language development and difficulty expressing needs
- Laughing or crying for no apparent reason
- Indifference toward others, dislike of touching and cuddling, lack of eye contact
- Intense need for routine and dislike of change
- Self-injurious behaviors, such as head banging, hitting, or biting; no fear of danger
- Repetitive rocking motions; hand flapping
- Frequent outbursts and tantrums

How it's treated

- Early intervention and special education programs to increase the child's capacity to learn, to facilitate his ability to communicate and relate to others, and to reduce disruptive behaviors
- Family education and counseling

- In some cases, stimulants, selective serotonin reuptake inhibitors, lithium, risperidone, or buspirone

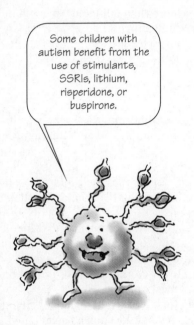

Basal cell carcinoma

- Slow-growing, destructive skin tumor; also called *basal cell epithelioma*
- Accounts for more than 50% of all cancers
- Diminished maturation and normal keratinization caused by changes in epidermal basal cells; mass formation caused by continuing division of basal cells

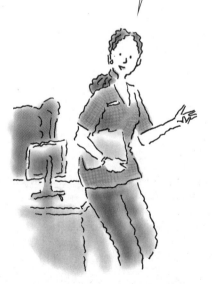

Basal cell carcinomas are destructive skin tumors. They account for more than 50% of all cancers.

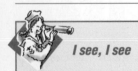

I see, I see

How basal cell carcinoma develops

Basal cell carcinoma is thought to originate when undifferentiated basal cells become carcinomatous instead of differentiating into sweat glands, sebum, and hair. The most common cancer, it begins as a papule, enlarges, and develops a central crater. Usually, this cancer spreads only locally.

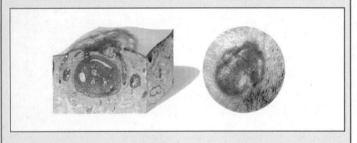

What causes it

- Most common: prolonged sun exposure
- Rare: arsenic, radiation exposure, burns, immunosuppression, vaccinations

What to look for

- Noduloulcerative lesions
  - Appear most commonly on the face (forehead, eyelid margins, nasolabial folds)
  - Early stages: small, smooth, pinkish and translucent papules; telangiectiatic vessels across the surface; lesions may be pigmented
  - As lesions enlarge: depressed center with firm, elevated borders

- – Ulceration and local invasion: eventually, chronic, persisting ulcers that spread locally but rarely metastasize
- – If left untreated, possibly spread to vital areas and become infected; may cause hemorrhage with invasion of large blood vessels

Whenever I'm at the beach, I make sure to put on sunscreen to protect myself from the sun's harmful rays!

- Superficial basal cell carcinoma
  - – Multiple lesions on the chest and back
  - – Oval or irregularly shaped, lightly pigmented plaques with sharply defined, slightly elevated, threadlike borders
  - – Superficial erosion: lesions appear scaly, with small atrophic areas in the center that resemble psoriasis or eczema
- Sclerosis basal cell carcinoma
  - – Occur on the head and neck
  - – Lesions appear as waxy, sclerotic, yellow to white plaques that resemble scar tissue without distinct borders

How it's treated

- Curettage and electrodesiccation to remove small lesions (good cosmetic results)
- Topical fluorouracil to treat superficial lesions (causing marked local irritation or inflammation but no systemic effects)
- Microscopically controlled surgical excision to carefully remove recurrent lesions until tumor-free plane is achieved

(skin grafting possibly necessary after removal of large lesions)
- Irradiation to eradicate tumor (depending on tumor location and if patient is elderly or debilitated and unable to withstand surgery)
- Cryotherapy (with liquid nitrogen) to freeze and kill cancerous cells
- Chemosurgery to kill cancer cells (possibly necessary for persistent or recurrent lesions)
- Avoidance of excessive sun exposure and use of sunscreen or sunshade to protect the skin from ultraviolet rays
- Regular follow-up care for screening and lifelong vigilance against recurrence, even after successful treatment

Bipolar disorder

- Marked by severe, pathologic mood swings from hyperactivity and euphoria to sadness and depression
- Type I: alternating episodes of mania and depression
- Type II: recurrent depressive episodes and occasional mild manic (hypomanic) episodes
- Seasonal pattern: onset of the mood episode occurs during a particular 60-day period of the year

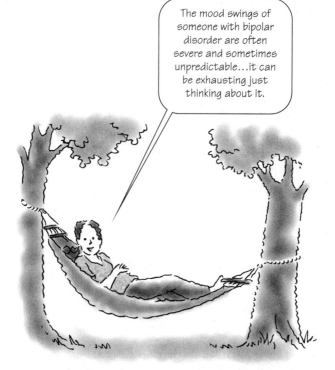

What causes it
- No clear cause (hereditary, biological, and psychological factors may play a part)
- Emotional or physical trauma preceding the disorder

What to look for

Manic episode
- Grandiose, euphoric appearance
- Irritability, with little control over activities and responses
- Hyperactive or excessive behavior
- Inflated sense of self-esteem, which may be delusional
- Accelerated and pressured speech
- Flight of ideas and easy distractibility
- Signs of malnutrition and poor personal hygiene

Hypomanic episode
- Euphoric but unstable mood
- Pressured speech
- Increased motor activity

Depressive episode
- Loss of self-esteem
- Sense of overwhelming inertia
- Social withdrawal
- Hopelessness, apathy, or self-reproach
- Slow speech and response
- Subjective difficulty concentrating or thinking clearly
- Headache
- Lethargy; slow gait and low muscle tone
- Weight loss and constipation
- Sleep disturbances
- Sexual dysfunction
- Chest pain
- Hypochondria
- Suicidal ideation, possibly with homicidal ideation

How it's treated

- Lithium to relieve and prevent manic episodes
- Anticonvulsants, either alone or with lithium
- Electroconvulsive therapy to treat severe depression
- Antidepressants (may trigger a manic episode)
- Careful monitoring for side effects and toxicity from medications
- Ongoing evaluation of treatment, disorder status, and self-care ability

Bladder cancer

- May develop on surface of bladder wall (benign or malignant papillomas) or grow within bladder wall (generally more virulent) and quickly invade underlying muscles
- Most common type: transitional cell carcinoma, arising from transitional epithelium of mucous membranes
- Less common types: adenocarcinomas, epidermoid carcinomas, squamous cell carcinomas, sarcomas, tumors in bladder diverticula, and carcinoma in situ
- Early stages commonly asymptomatic

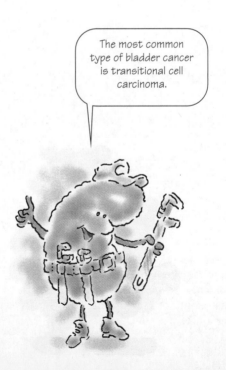

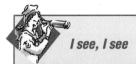

I see, I see

How bladder cancer develops

Bladder tumors can develop on the surface of the bladder wall or grow within the bladder wall and quickly invade underlying muscle. Most bladder tumors (90%) are transitional cell carcinomas, arising from the transitional epithelium of mucous membranes. They may also result from malignant transformation of benign papillomas. This illustration shows a bladder carcinoma infiltrating the bladder wall.

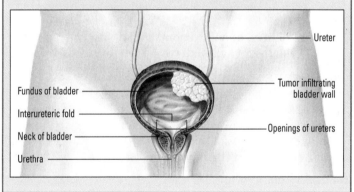

What causes it

- Primary cause unknown

Risk factors

- Environmental carcinogens (smoking, arsenic, 2-naphthy-lamine, nitrates)
- Family history of bladder cancer
- Schistosomiasis (squamous cell carcinoma of bladder; most common in endemic areas)
- Chronic bladder irritation and infection, history of kidney or bladder stones, limited fluid intake

What to look for
- Gross, painless, intermittent hematuria, frequently with clots
- Suprapubic pain after voiding
- Bladder irritability, urinary frequency, nocturia, dribbling

How it's treated

Superficial bladder tumors
- Transurethral (cystoscopic) resection and fulguration (electrical destruction) to remove tumor
- Intravesicular chemotherapy (for multiple tumors) to kill cancer cells
- Fulguration if additional tumors develop (may be repeated every 3 months for years) to remove tumor

Large tumor
- Segmental bladder resection to remove full-thickness section of bladder (only if tumor isn't near bladder neck or ureteral orifices)
- Bladder instillations of thiotepa after transurethral resection to slow or stop growth of cancer cells

Infiltrating bladder tumors
- Radical cystectomy
  - Treatment of choice for infiltrating bladder tumors
  - Requires urinary diversion (usually ileal conduit)
- Possible penile implant (later) to treat erectile dysfunction
- Referral to American Cancer Society or United Ostomy Association (if patient received ostomy) for information and support

Advanced bladder cancer
- Cystectomy to remove tumor
- Radiation therapy to destroy cancer cells

- Systemic chemotherapy (cisplatin, cyclophosphamide, fluorouracil, doxorubicin) to destroy cancer cells
- Investigational treatments (clinical trials currently being conducted)
  - Photodynamic therapy and intravesicular administration of interferon alfa and tumor necrosis factor to destroy cancer cells
  - Bacille Calmette-Guérin (immunomodulating agent) to treat superficial bladder cancer after surgery to remove tumor
  - Biological response modifiers (interferons, interleukins, colony-stimulating factors, monoclonal antibodies, vaccines) to destroy cancer cells

Breast cancer

- Most common cancer affecting women (less than 1% incidence in men)
- Commonly develops after age 50

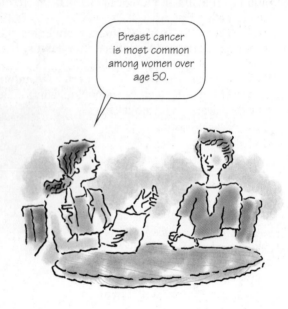

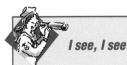

I see, I see

Cellular progression of breast cancer

Breast cancer growth rates vary. It spreads by way of the lymphatic system and bloodstream to the other breast, chest wall, liver, bone, and brain.

Classification of breast cancer is usually made according to histologic appearance and the lesion's location:

- *adenocarcinoma*—arising from the epithelium
- *intraductal*—developing within the ducts (includes Paget's disease)
- *infiltrating*—occurring in parenchymal tissue
- *inflammatory* (rare)—rapidly growing and causing overlying skin to become edematous, inflamed, and indurated
- *lobular carcinoma in situ*—involving lobes of glandular tissue
- *medullary* or *circumscribed*—enlarging rapidly.

Breast cancer originates in the epithelial lining of the breast. This illustration shows the intraductal changes, with transformation of benign cells to atypical cells to malignant cells.

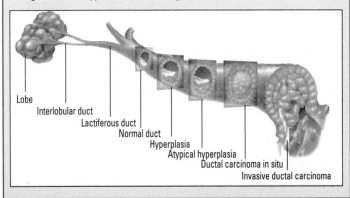

Lobe
Interlobular duct
Lactiferous duct
Normal duct
Hyperplasia
Atypical hyperplasia
Ductal carcinoma in situ
Invasive ductal carcinoma

What causes it

- No proven cause (estrogen is implicated because of high incidence of breast cancer in women)
- Possible causes
  - Estrogen therapy
  - Antihypertensive agents
  - High-fat diet
  - Obesity
  - Fibrocystic breast disease

Risk factors

- Factors associated with higher risk
  - Family history of breast cancer, particularly first-degree relative (mother or sister)
  - Genetic mutations in BRCA1 and BRCA2 genes (suggesting genetic predisposition)
  - Long menses (menses beginning early or menopause beginning late)
  - No history of pregnancy
  - First pregnancy after age 30
  - History of unilateral breast cancer (high risk of recurrence)
  - History of endometrial or ovarian cancer
  - Exposure to low-level ionizing radiation
- Factors associated with lower risk
  - History of pregnancy before age 20
  - History of multiple pregnancies
  - Native American or Asian ethnicity

What to look for

- Lump or mass in the breast (a hard, stony mass is usually malignant)
- Change in symmetry or size of the breast
- Change in skin: Peau d'orange (edematous thickening and pitting), scaly skin around the nipple, or ulceration
- Warm, hot or pink area on the breast

- Unusual discharge or drainage—spontaneous or expressed
- Change in nipple, such as itching, burning, erosion, or retraction
- Pain (usually in advanced stages)
- Bone metastasis, pathologic bone fractures, and hypercalcemia
- Arm edema

How it's treated

Surgery

- Lumpectomy (may be combined with radiation therapy), lumpectomy and dissection of axillary lymph nodes, simple mastectomy, modified radical mastectomy, or radical mastectomy to remove diseased tissue
- Reconstructive surgery (after mastectomy) to restore normal anatomical appearance and improve self-esteem

Medicine

- Chemotherapy (cyclophosphamide, fluorouracil, methotrexate, doxorubicin, vincristine, paclitaxel, prednisone) to kill cancer cells
- Antiestrogens (tamoxifen, fulvestrant, toremifene) to bind to estrogen receptors, block estrogen action, and inhibit estrogen-mediated tumor growth in breast tissue
- Aromatase inhibitors (anastrozole, letrozole) to treat metastatic breast cancer in postmenopausal women

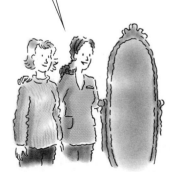

Reconstructive surgery can help restore a more normal appearance to your breast after a mastectomy.

- Monoclonal antibody immunotherapy (trastuzumab) to treat women whose cancer tests positive for HER2/neu and to treat cancer that returns or progresses during chemotherapy
- Peripheral stem cell therapy to treat advanced breast cancer
- Primary radiation therapy for small tumors in early stages with no evidence of distant metastasis; also used to prevent or treat local recurrence
- Presurgical radiation (in patients with inflammatory breast cancer) to help make tumors more surgically manageable
- Palliative treatment (pain management, radiation therapy) for bone metastasis to maintain comfort

Other measures

- Referral to American Cancer Society's Reach to Recovery program to provide instruction, emotional support, counseling, and information about breast prostheses
- Information about breast cancer detection, monthly breast self-examination, and professional clinical breast examinations and mammography, according to the American Cancer Society guidelines

Bronchiectasis

- Chronic abnormal dilation of bronchi and destruction of bronchial walls
- Can occur throughout tracheobronchial tree or be confined to a single segment or lobe
- Usually bilateral, involving basilar segments of lower lobes
- Three forms of bronchiectasis: cylindrical, fusiform (varicose), and saccular (cystic)

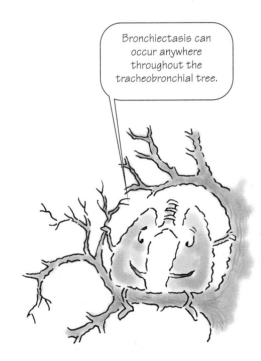

Bronchiectasis can occur anywhere throughout the tracheobronchial tree.

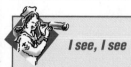

I see, I see

How bronchiectasis develops

Injury to bronchial walls

⬇

Replacement of damaged lining with hyperplastic squamous epithelium that lacks cilia to move secretions

⬇

Stagnation of sputum, leading to dilation of bronchial airways and secondary infections

⬇

Inflammation and accumulation of secretions

⬇

Further mucosal injury due to pressure from retained secretions

⬇

Bronchial dilation and scarring, altering airflow to lungs and increasing risk of infection

⬇

Additional damage and progression of disease (a form of chronic obstructive pulmonary disease) with each subsequent infection

What causes it

- Cystic fibrosis
- Immunologic disorders, such as agammaglobulinemia
- Recurrent, inadequately treated bacterial respiratory tract infections, such as tuberculosis
- Measles, pneumonia, pertussis, or influenza
- Obstruction by a foreign body, tumor, or stenosis associated with recurrent infection
- Inhalation of corrosive gas or repeated aspiration of gastric juices

What to look for

- Possibly no symptoms initially
- Chronic cough with copious, foul-smelling, mucopurulent secretions
- Hemoptysis
- Coarse crackles during inspiration over involved lung areas
- Occasional wheezes
- Dyspnea
- Weight loss, malnutrition, anemia, malaise
- Clubbing
- Recurrent fever, chills, and other signs of infection
- Right-sided heart failure and cor pulmonale in advanced cases

How it's treated

- Antibiotics to treat recurrent infections
- Bronchodilators, with postural drainage and chest percussion, to help remove secretions
- Bronchoscopy to aid in removal of secretions in severe cases
- Oxygen therapy to treat hypoxia
- Lobectomy or segmental resection for severe hemoptysis
- Supportive nutrition and adequate hydration
- Smoking cessation to decrease irritation
- Avoidance of respiratory irritants, crowds, and people with respiratory tract infections
- Pneumococcal and influenza immunizations

Bronchitis

- Form of chronic obstructive pulmonary disease
- Characterized by excessive production of tracheobronchial mucus and chronic cough (at least 3 months each year for 2 consecutive years)
- Distinguishing characteristic: airflow obstruction

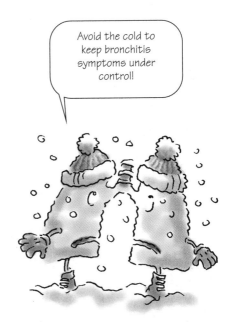

What causes it

- Cigarette smoking
- Genetic predisposition
- Organic or inorganic dusts and noxious gas exposure
- Respiratory tract infection

What to look for

- Productive cough with copious gray, white, or yellow sputum
- Dyspnea
- Tachypnea, cyanosis, and use of accessory muscles for breathing
- Wheezing and rhonchi
- Prolonged expiration
- Pedal edema and jugular vein distention with right-sided heart failure

This is intense

Acute respiratory failure

Acute respiratory failure in the patient with chronic bronchitis is an emergency. If your patient's respiratory status deteriorates, proceed as follows:

• Administer an antibiotic, a bronchodilator, an anxiolytic, and, possibly, a steroid, as ordered.
• Administer oxygen and monitor for improved breathing.
• For significant respiratory acidosis, a bidirectional positive-pressure airway mask or mechanical ventilation through an endotracheal or tracheostomy tube may be necessary.
• Encourage the patient to cough and deep-breathe with pursed lips.
• If the patient is alert, have him use an incentive spirometer; if he's intubated and lethargic, turn him every 1 to 2 hours.
• Use postural drainage and chest physiotherapy to help clear the patient's secretions.
• If the patient is intubated, suction his trachea. Observe him for a change in the quantity, consistency, or color of his sputum. Provide humidification to liquefy the secretions.
• Observe the patient closely for respiratory arrest. Auscultate for breath sounds and monitor arterial blood gases for changes.
• Monitor serum electrolyte levels and correct imbalances.
• Monitor intake and output and daily weight.
• Monitor for cardiac arrhythmias.

How it's treated

• Antibiotics to treat recurring infections
• Bronchodilators to relieve bronchospasms and facilitate mucociliary clearance
• Adequate hydration to liquefy secretions
• Chest physiotherapy to mobilize secretions

- Ultrasonic or mechanical nebulizers to loosen and mobilize secretions
- Corticosteroids to combat inflammation
- Diuretics to reduce edema
- Oxygen to treat hypoxia
- Smoking cessation and avoidance of air pollutants to decrease irritation
- Avoidance of blasts of cold air, which can precipitate bronchospasm
- Avoidance of crowds and people with known respiratory tract infections
- Pneumococcal and influenza immunizations

Buerger's disease

- Inflammatory, nonatheromatous occlusive condition
- Circulation impairment to the legs, feet, and occasionally the hands
- Causes segmental lesions and subsequent thrombus formation in small and medium arteries and sometimes in the veins
- Affected arteries prone to spasms, which constrict the arterial lumen

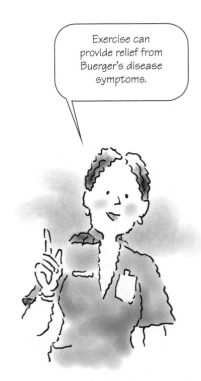

Exercise can provide relief from Buerger's disease symptoms.

What causes it

- Unknown cause
- Linked to smoking, suggesting a hypersensitivity reaction to nicotine
- May be associated with Raynaud's disease and may occur in people with autoimmune disease

What to look for

- Intermittent claudication of the instep, aggravated by exercise and relieved by rest
- Feet that initially become cold, cyanotic, and numb after exposure to cold and later redden, become hot, and tingle
- Impaired peripheral pulses
- Migratory superficial thrombophlebitis
- Limb pain, ulceration, gangrene

How it's treated

- Aspirin and vasodilator to promote circulation
- Exercise program that uses gravity to fill and drain blood vessels to relieve symptoms
- Lumbar sympathectomy to increase blood supply to the skin in severe cases
- Amputation for nonhealing ulcers, intractable pain, or gangrene
- Smoking cessation
- Proper foot care for ulcer prevention
- Avoidance of precipitating factors, such as emotional stress, exposure to extreme temperatures, and trauma

Bulimia nervosa

- Eating disorder marked by episodes of binge eating followed by feelings of guilt, humiliation, depression, and self-condemnation
- Impulsive, excessive eating of restricted foods followed by panic that food will turn to fat
- Binges tending to occur several times a day, generally after an extended period of dieting
- Use of measures to prevent weight gain (self-induced vomiting, use of diuretics or laxatives, dieting, fasting)

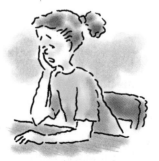

People with bulimia nervosa commonly experience feelings of guilt, humiliation, depression, and self-condemnation after episodes of bingeing and purging.

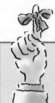

Memory jogger

Although not all bulimics engage in purging, the term RIDS BODY can help you remember the clinical features of bulimia.

R Recurrent binge-eating episodes

I Intense exercise

D Diuretic, laxative, or enema use

S Self-induced vomiting

B Body image distortion

O Ordinary eating alternating with episodes of bingeing and purging

D Depression and anxiety disorders possible

Y Yo-yo effect of tension relief and pleasure experienced with bingeing; guilt and depression after purging

What causes it

- No proven cause
- Contributing factors: genetic, biological, behavioral, environmental, family, and psychosocial elements (such as family conflict, sexual abuse, maladaptive learned behavior, and struggle for control or identity)

What to look for

Physical findings

- Thin, normal, or slightly overweight appearance
- Frequent weight fluctuations
- Persistent sore throat and heartburn, salivary gland swelling, hoarseness, throat lacerations, and dental erosion (from vomiting)
- Calluses or scarring on the back of hands and knuckles (from inducing vomiting)

- Abdominal and epigastric pain
- Amenorrhea

Psychosocial findings

- Perfectionism
- Distorted body image
- Exaggerated sense of guilt
- Feelings of alienation, impaired social or occupational adjustment
- Recurrent anxiety
- Depression, self-consciousness
- Poor impulse control
- Low tolerance for frustration
- Difficulty expressing such feelings as anger
- History of childhood trauma
- History of unsatisfactory sexual relationships
- Parental obesity

Behavioral findings

- Evidence of binge eating (disappearance of large amounts of food; presence of large number of food containers or wrappers)
- Evidence of purging (frequent trips to the bathroom after meals; presence of packages of diuretics and laxatives)
- Peculiar eating habits or rituals
- Excessive, rigid exercise regimen
- Complex schedule to make time for binge-and-purge sessions
- Withdrawal from friends and usual activities
- Hyperactivity
- Frequent weighing

How it's treated

- Treatment centered on cause and including individual, group, and family therapy
- Nutrition counseling

- Medications such as tricyclic antidepressants or selective serotonin reuptake inhibitors
- Possible hospitalization based on the patient's physical condition and need for observation
- Early treatment crucial before behaviors become ingrained

C–G

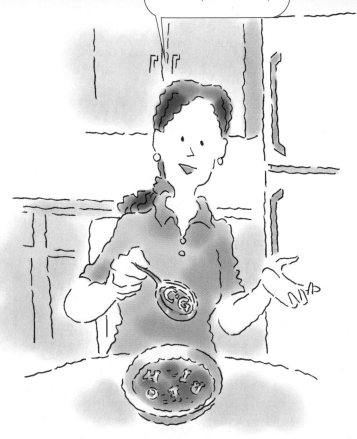

Cardiomyopathy, dilated

- Disease of heart muscle fibers
- Usually not diagnosed until advanced stage; prognosis generally poor
- Leads to intractable heart failure, arrhythmias, and emboli

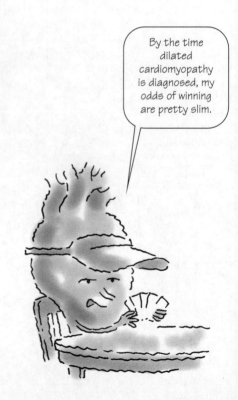

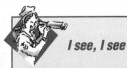

I see, I see

Understanding dilated cardiomyopathy

In dilated cardiomyopathy, extensively damaged myocardial muscle fibers reduce contractility of the left ventricle. As systolic function declines, stroke volume, ejection fraction, and cardiac output fall. The sympathetic nervous system is stimulated to increase heart rate and contractility. The kidneys are stimulated to retain sodium and water to maintain cardiac output, and vasoconstriction also occurs as the renin-angiotensin system is stimulated.

When compensatory mechanisms can no longer maintain cardiac output, the heart begins to fail. Left ventricular dilation occurs as venous return and systemic vascular resistance rise. Eventually, the atria also dilate as more work is required to pump blood into the full ventricles. Cardiomegaly occurs due to dilation of the atria and ventricles.

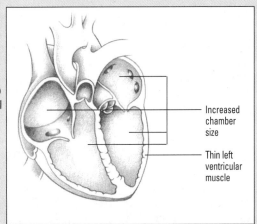

Increased chamber size

Thin left ventricular muscle

What causes it

- Idiopathic
- Myocarditis
- Viral or bacterial infections

- Hypertension
- Peripartum syndrome related to pregnancy-induced hypertension
- Ischemic heart disease
- Valvular disease
- Drug hypersensitivity
- Chemotherapy
- Cardiotoxic effects of drug or alcohol

What to look for

- Left-sided heart failure
  - Shortness of breath
  - Orthopnea and paroxysmal nocturnal dypsnea
  - Dyspnea on exertion
  - Dizziness
  - Fatigue
  - Dry cough
- Right-sided heart failure
  - Peripheral edema
  - Hepatomegaly
  - Jugular vein distention
  - Weight gain
- Low cardiac output
  - Peripheral cyanosis
  - Tachycardia
  - Decreased renal perfusion and renal failure
- Murmur from mitral and tricuspid insufficiency due to cardiomegaly and weak papillary muscles
- S_3 and S_4 gallop due to heart failure
- Atrial fibrillation

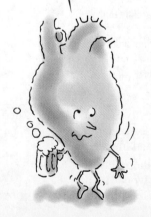

Go easy on the alcohol. The toxic effects of excessive drinking can lead me to fail.

How it's treated

- ACE inhibitors to reduce afterload through vasodilation
- Diuretics to reduce fluid retention; potassium supplements as needed
- Digoxin and dobutamine to improve myocardial contractility for a patient who doesn't respond to diuretics
- Hydralazine and isosorbide dinitrate to produce vasodilation
- Beta-adrenergic blockers to treat New York Heart Association (NYHA) class II or III heart failure
- Antiarrhythmics, pacemaker, or implantable cardioverter-defibrillator (ICD) to control arrhythmias
- Anticoagulants to prevent clot formation
- Biventricular pacemaker for cardiac resynchronization therapy (if symptoms continue despite optimal drug therapy, QRS duration is 0.12 second or more, or ejection fraction is 35% or less, the patient is classified as NYHA class III or IV heart failure)
- Revascularization (such as CABG surgery) to manage dilated cardiomyopathy from ischemia
- Valvular repair or replacement to manage dilated cardiomyopathy from valve dysfunction
- Heart transplantation for patient who doesn't respond to other medical therapy
- Lifestyle modifications (smoking cessation; low-fat, low-sodium diet; physical activity; abstinence from alcohol) to reduce symptoms and improve quality of life

You won't find triple chocolate swirl on the dietary recommendations for a patient with dilated cardiomyopathy.

Cardiomyopathy, hypertrophic obstructive

- Also called IHSS (idiopathic hypertrophic subaortic stenosis)
- Primary disease of cardiac muscle and intraventricular septum
- 50% of all sudden deaths in competitive athletes are due to hypertrophic obstructive cardiomyopathy (HOCM)

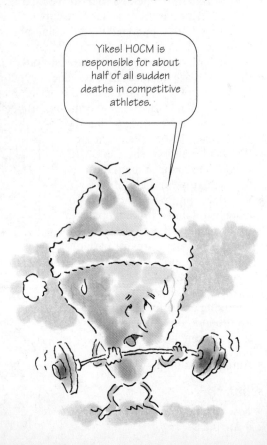

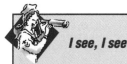

I see, I see

Understanding HOCM

HOCM affects diastolic function. The left ventricle and intraventricular septum hypertrophy and become stiff, noncompliant, and unable to relax during ventricular filling. Ventricular filling decreases and left ventricular filling pressure rises, causing a rise in left atrial and pulmonary venous pressures. This rise in pressure leads to rapid, forceful contractions of the left ventricle and impaired relaxation. The forceful ejection of blood draws the anterior leaflet of the mitral valve to the intraventricular septum, which causes early closure of the outflow tract, decreasing ejection fraction.

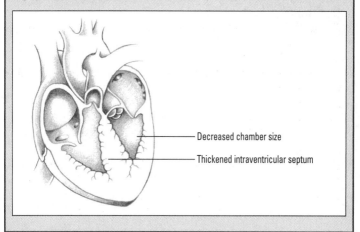

Decreased chamber size

Thickened intraventricular septum

What causes it
• Autosomal dominant trait

What to look for
• Low cardiac output
  – Angina pectoris

  – Arrhythmias, atrial fibrillation
  – Dyspnea, orthopnea
  – Fatigue
  – Syncope
  – Heart failure
- Harsh mid-systolic ejection murmur
- Pulsus bisferiens

How it's treated

- Beta-adrenergic blockers to slow heart rate, reduce myocardial oxygen demands, and increase ventricular filling by relaxing obstructing muscle, thereby increasing cardiac output
- Antiarrhythmic drugs, such as amiodarone, to reduce arrhythmias
- Cardioversion to treat atrial fibrillation
- Anticoagulation to reduce risk of systemic embolism with atrial fibrillation
- Calcium channel blockers to reduce septal stiffness and elevated diastolic pressures
- ICD to treat ventricular arrhythmias
- Ventricular myotomy or myectomy (resection of hypertrophied septum) to ease outflow tract obstruction and relieve symptoms
- Prophylactic antibiotics before dental work or invasive procedures
- Family screening due to genetic component

Cardiomyopathy, restrictive

- Disease of heart muscle fibers
- Irreversible if severe

I see, I see

Understanding restrictive cardiomyopathy

Restrictive cardiomyopathy is characterized by stiffness of the ventricle caused by left ventricular hypertrophy and endocardial fibrosis and thickening, which reduces the ventricle's ability to relax and fill during diastole. The rigid myocardium fails to contract completely during systole. As a result, cardiac output falls.

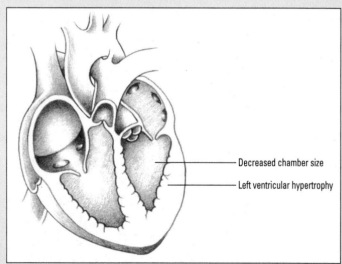

Decreased chamber size

Left ventricular hypertrophy

What causes it

- Amyloidosis
- Sarcoidosis
- Hemochromatosis
- Infiltrative neoplastic disease

What to look for

- Decreased cardiac output
  - Heart failure, generalized edema, liver engorgement
  - Fatigue
  - Dyspnea, orthopnea
  - Chest pain
  - Peripheral cyanosis, pallor
  - S_3 or S_4 gallop
- Murmur due to mitral and tricuspid insufficiency

How it's treated

- Supportive treatment of the underlying disorder
- Digoxin, diuretics, and restricted sodium diet to ease symptoms of heart failure
- Oral vasodilators to decrease afterload and facilitate ventricular ejection
- Anticoagulant therapy to prevent clot formation due to decreased cardiac output and immobility from exercise intolerance
- Deferoxamine to bind iron in restrictive cardiomyopathy due to hemochromatosis

Carpal tunnel syndrome

- Compression of median nerve as it passes through canal (tunnel) formed by carpal bones and transverse carpal ligaments
- Most common nerve entrapment syndrome

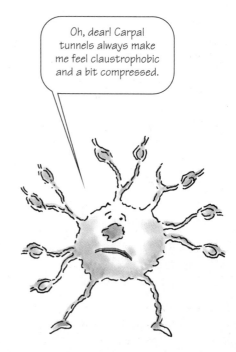

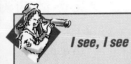

I see, I see

Understanding carpal tunnel syndrome

Compression of the median nerve causes sensory and motor changes in the hand's median distribution, impairing sensory transmission to the thumb, index and second fingers, and inner aspect of the third finger.

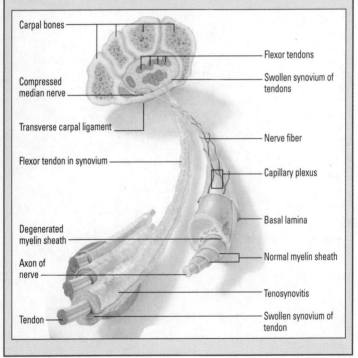

Carpal bones

Compressed median nerve

Transverse carpal ligament

Flexor tendon in synovium

Degenerated myelin sheath

Axon of nerve

Tendon

Flexor tendons

Swollen synovium of tendons

Nerve fiber

Capillary plexus

Basal lamina

Normal myelin sheath

Tenosynovitis

Swollen synovium of tendon

What causes it
- Congenital predisposition
- Trauma or injury to wrist

- Overactive pituitary gland
- Thyroid disorder
- Rheumatoid arthritis or osteoarthritis
- Mechanical problems in wrist joint
- Work-related stress, such as repetitive tasks with forceful flexion and extension of the tendons of the wrist and hand
- Fluid retention during pregnancy or menopause
- Development of cyst or tumor within canal
- Obesity

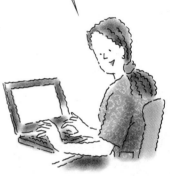

This typing is killing my median nerve. I gotta take a break!

What to look for

- Weakness, pain, burning, numbness, or tingling in the hands
- Affects the thumb, forefinger, middle finger, and half of the fourth finger
- Inability to clench a fist
- Atrophic nails
- Symptoms that worsen at night
- May spread to the forearm and, in severe cases, to the shoulder or neck

How it's treated

- Splinting wrist in neutral extension for 1 to 2 weeks to rest hand
- Nonsteroidal anti-inflammatory drugs (NSAIDs) to relieve symptoms
- Injection of carpal tunnel with hydrocortisone and lidocaine to provide significant but temporary relief of symptoms
- Surgical decompression of nerve (resection of entire transverse carpal tunnel ligament or endoscopic techniques) to relieve compression on the nerve

- Occupational therapy and ergonomic assessment of the work environment (for those who must remain in current occupation) or job retraining (if link to job has been established) to prevent recurrence of symptoms

Celiac disease

- Also known as idiopathic steatorrhea, nontropical sprue, gluten enteropathy and celiac sprue
- Poor food absorption and intolerance of gluten, a protein in wheat and wheat products
- Malabsorption in small bowel, which results from atrophy of the villi and decreased activity and amount of enzymes

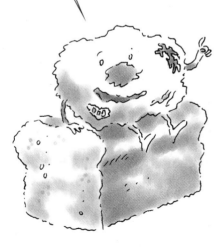

What causes it
- Environmental factors
- Genetic predisposition
- May also be autoimmune

What to look for
- GI
  - Diarrhea, steatorrhea, stomach cramps
  - Abdominal distention and flatulence
  - Anorexia, or occasionally increased appetite without weight gain
  - Weakness and weight loss
- Musculoskeletal
  - Osteomalacia, osteoporosis
  - Tetany
  - Bone pain
- Neurologic
  - Peripheral neuropathy
  - Seizures
  - Parethesia
- Dermatologic
  - Dry skin and brittle nails
  - Fine, sparse, prematurely gray hair
  - Eczema, psoriasis, dermatitis herpetiformis and acne roacea
  - Localized hyperpigmentation on the face, lips, or mucosa
- Endocrine
  - Amenorrhea
  - Hypometabolism
  - Adrenocortical insufficiency
- Psychosocial
  - Mood changes and irritability
- Hematologic
  - Anemia
  - Hypoprothrombinemia and risk of bleeding

How it's treated

- Elimination of gluten (wheat, barley, rye, and oat products) from the diet for life
- Dietary supplements including iron, vitamin B_{12}, folic acid, and vitamin K
- Electrolyte and fluid replacement to counter diarrhea
- Corticosteroid for adrenal insufficiency

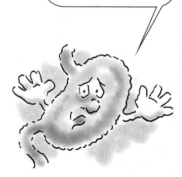

Cerebral palsy

- Group of neuromuscular disorders resulting from prenatal, perinatal, or postnatal central nervous system damage
- Nonprogressive disorder of three major types, which may be combined
  - Spastic: cortex is affected
  - Athetoid: basal ganglia are injured
  - Ataxic: cerebellum is affected
- Motor impairment may be minimal or severely disabling with associated defects, such as seizures, speech disorders, and mental retardation

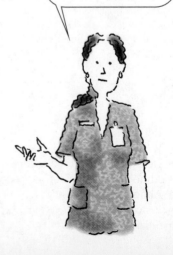

Some patients with cerebral palsy have minimal motor impairment, whereas others are severely disabled.

What causes it

- Conditions that result in cerebral anoxia, hemorrhage, or other damage

---

Causes of cerebral palsy

Conditions that result in cerebral anoxia, hemorrhage, or other damage are probably responsible for cerebral palsy (CP):

- *Prenatal conditions that may increase risk of CP:* maternal infection (especially rubella), maternal drug ingestion, radiation, anoxia, toxemia, maternal diabetes, abnormal placental attachment, malnutrition, and isoimmunization
- *Perinatal and birth difficulties that increase the risk of CP:* forceps delivery, breech presentation, placenta previa, abruptio placentae, metabolic or electrolyte disturbances, abnormal maternal vital signs from general or spinal anesthetic, prolapsed cord with delay in delivery of head, premature birth, prolonged or unusually rapid labor, and multiple birth (especially infants born last in a multiple birth)
- *Infection or trauma during infancy:* poisoning, severe kernicterus resulting from erythroblastosis fetalis, brain infection, head trauma, prolonged anoxia, brain tumor, cerebral circulatory anomalies causing blood vessel rupture, and systemic disease resulting in cerebral thrombosis or embolus.

What to look for

- Excessive lethargy or irritability
- High-pitched cry
- Poor head control
- Weak sucking reflex
- Delayed motor development
- Abnormal head circumference (typically smaller)
- Abnormal postures, reflexes, and muscle tone
- Vision and hearing deficits
- Seizure activity

How it's treated

- Supportive care including physical and occupational therapy and assistive devices to maximize abilities and independence
- Orthopedic surgery or botulinum toxin to treat contractures
- Anticonvulsants to control seizures
- Muscle relaxants or neurosurgery to decrease spasticity

Cervical cancer

- Preinvasive
  - Ranges from minimal cervical dysplasia to carcinoma in situ
  - Generally curable with early detection and treatment
- Invasive
  - Penetration of basement membrane by cancer cells, which spread directly to adjoining pelvic structures or systemically by the lymphatic route

What causes it

- Unknown cause
- Predisposing factors
  - Frequent intercourse at a young age (under 16 years old)
  - Multiple sexual partners
  - Multiple pregnancies
  - Exposure to sexually transmitted diseases, particularly genital human papillomavirus
  - Smoking

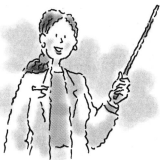

Women of reproductive age should have a Pap smear annually.

What to look for

- Preinvasive cervical carcinoma: no symptoms
- Invasive cervical carcinoma: abnormal vaginal bleeding and persistent discharge, postcoital pain and bleeding
- Advanced invasive cervical carcinoma: pelvic pain, vaginal leakage of urine and feces from fistulas, anorexia, weight loss, and anemia
- Positive Papanicolaou smear
- Other positive follow-up studies, such as colposcopy, lymphangiography, and cystography

How it's treated

- Preinvasive cervical cancer: total excisional biopsy, cryosurgery, laser destruction, conization with frequent Pap smear follow-up, or, rarely, hysterectomy
- Invasive squamous cell cancer: radical hysterectomy, radiation therapy (internal and external), and chemotherapy used in combination, depending on the cancer stage

Head of the class

Cervical cancer prevention: The HPV vaccine

Due to the high risk of cervical cancer following infection with human papillomavirus (HPV), the HPV vaccine is recommended for women 26 years old or younger. Ideally, the vaccine should be administered before potential exposure to HPV through sexual activity. Routine vaccination is recommended for females aged 11 to 12 years but can be started as young as age 9. Unvaccinated females aged 13 to 26 years should receive catch-up vaccinations. Although the vaccination is less beneficial for women who have already been infected with one or more of the four HPV types, sexually active women should still be vaccinated.

Cholelithiasis

- Stone or calculi (gallstones) in the gallbladder

I see, I see

Understanding gallstone formation

Abnormal metabolism of cholesterol and bile salts plays an important role in gallstone formation. The liver makes bile continuously. The gall bladder concentrates and stores it until the duodenum signals it needs it to help digest fat. Changes in the composition of bile may allow gallstones to form. Changes to the absorptive ability of the gallbladder lining may also contribute to gallstone formation.

Certain conditions, such as age, obesity, and estrogen imbalance, cause the liver to secrete bile that's abnormally high in cholesterol or lacking the proper concentration of bile salts.

When the gallbladder concentrates this bile, inflammation may occur. Excessive reabsorption of water and bile salts makes the bile less soluble. Cholesterol, calcium, and bilirubin precipitate into gallstones.

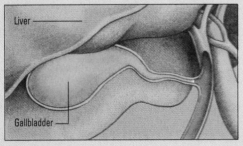

Liver

Gallbladder

What causes it

- Changes in bile components during periods of sluggishness in the gallbladder
  - Pregnancy
  - Hormonal contraceptive use
  - Diabetes mellitus
  - Celiac disease
  - Cirrhosis of the liver
  - Pancreatitis

What to look for

- May produce no symptoms
- Right upper quadrant pain with radiation to the back, between the shoulders, or to the front of the chest, mimicking chest pain
- Pain following meals rich in fats
- Pain at night that suddenly awakens the patient
- Belching, flatulence
- Indigestion, nausea, vomiting
- Low-grade fever, chills
- Jaundice if a stone obstructs the common bile duct
- Clay-colored stools

How it's treated

- Surgery (treatment of choice)
- Electrohydraulic shock wave lithotripsy to break up stones
- Percutaneous placement of a T-tube
- Ursodeoxycholic acid or chenodeoxycholic acid to dissolve stones
- Low-fat diet to alleviate symptoms
- Vitamin K supplement for itching, jaundice, and bleeding tendencies due to deficiency

Chronic fatigue syndrome

- May develop within a few hours and last for 6 months or more
- Common in females younger than age 45
- Marked by debilitating fatigue, neurologic abnormalities, and persistent symptoms

What causes it

- Unknown: possibly viral immune or autoimmune response

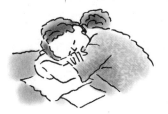

I just can't figure out why I'm so exhausted all the time!

What to look for

- Overwhelming fatigue unrelieved by rest and severe enough to restrict activities of daily living by half
- Fatigue not caused by exertion
- Headaches of a new pattern or severity
- Multiple joint pain without redness or swelling
- Muscle pain
- Postexertional malaise lasting 24 hours or longer
- Self-reported impairment in short-term memory
- Sore throat
- Tender cervical or axillary nodes
- Persistence of symptoms for 6 months or more

How it's treated

- Symptomatic care
- Medication to treat depression, anxiety, pain, and fever
- Antiviral drugs and selected immunomodulation agents to reduce symptoms
- Activity modification without becoming sedentary; exercise as tolerated
- Diet high in vitamins and minerals

Cirrhosis

- Chronic disease characterized by diffuse destruction and fibrotic regeneration of hepatic cells
- Damages liver tissue and normal vasculature

I see, I see

Understanding cirrhosis

Cirrhosis is a chronic liver disease characterized by widespread destruction of hepatic cells. The destroyed cells are replaced by fibrotic cells in a process called *fibrotic regeneration.* As necrotic tissue yields to fibrosis, regenerative nodules form, and the liver parenchyma undergo extensive and irreversible fibrotic changes. The disease alters normal liver structure and vasculature, impairs blood and lymphatic flow, and, ultimately, causes hepatic insufficiency.

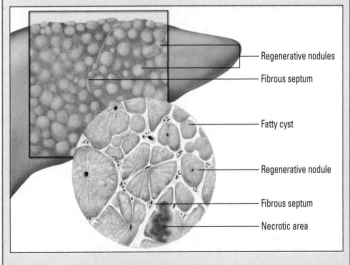

Regenerative nodules
Fibrous septum
Fatty cyst
Regenerative nodule
Fibrous septum
Necrotic area

What causes it
- Alcoholism
- Hepatitis
- Biliary obstruction
- Hemochromatosis
- Budd-Chiari syndrome (thrombosis of the hepatic vein)
- Alpha$_1$-antitrypsin deficiency
- Wilson's disease (disorder of copper metabolism)

What to look for
- Hepatomegaly
- Anorexia, nausea, vomiting, dull abdominal ache
- Edema and ascites
- Jaundice and dry skin
- Encephalopathy (lethargy, mental changes, slurred speech, peripheral neuritis, tremor)
- Bleeding tendencies and anemia
- Hypoxia due to pleural effusions and limited chest expansion from ascites
- Esophageal varices due to portal hypertension

How it's treated
- Cessation of alcohol ingestion to slow progression of disease
- Vitamins and nutritional supplements to improve nutritional status
- Potassium-sparing diuretics to reduce fluid accumulation
- Rest to conserve energy
- Vasopressin to treat esophageal varices
- Esophagogastric intubation with multilumen tubes to control bleeding from esophageal varices or other hemorrhage sites
- Paracentesis to relieve abdominal pressure and remove ascitic fluid
- Referral to Alcoholics Anonymous to provide support

- Lactulose to lower serum ammonia levels and treat encephalopathy
- Monitoring for coagulopathy and treatment with blood products or vitamin K as needed

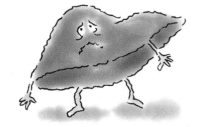

Colorectal cancer

- Slow-growing cancer that usually starts in the inner layer of the intestinal tract
- Commonly begins as a polyp
- Signs and symptoms dependent on tumor location
- Potentially curable if diagnosed early

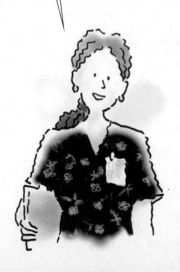

Colorectal cancer can be cured if it's diagnosed early and treated promptly.

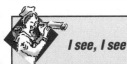

I see, I see

How colorectal cancer develops

Most lesions of the large bowel are moderately differentiated adenocarcinomas. These tumors tend to grow slowly and remain asymptomatic for long periods. Tumors in the rectum and sigmoid and descending colon grow circumferentially and constrict the intestinal lumen. Tumors in the ascending colon are usually large and palpable.

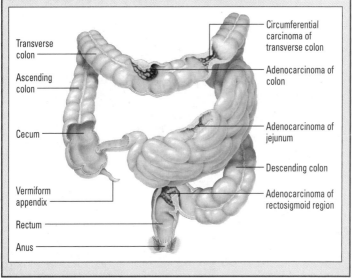

What causes it

- Exact cause unknown

Risk factors

- Inherited gene mutations
- Family or personal history of colorectal cancer
- History of intestinal polyps

- History of chronic inflammatory bowel disease
- Aging
- High-fat, low-fiber diet
- Obesity and physical inactivity
- Diabetes
- Smoking
- Heavy alcohol intake

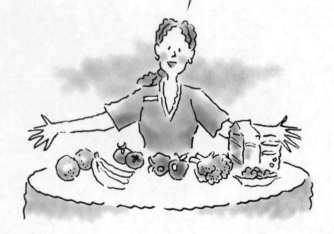

What to look for
- Depends on tumor location
- Black tarry stools to frank bleeding, possibly with mucus
- Signs and symptoms of intestinal obstruction: nausea, vomiting, anorexia, diarrhea, constipation, weight loss, ribbon- or pencil-shaped stools, pain relief from passage of stool or flatus
- Abdominal fullness, aching, cramps, rectal or sacral pressure
- Weakness, fatigue
- Exertional dyspnea
- Vertigo
- Palpable tumor

How it's treated
- Surgery to remove tumor
  - Right hemicolectomy (cecum and ascending colon)
  - Right colectomy (proximal and middle transverse colon)
  - Resection (typically limited to sigmoid colon)
  - Anterior or low anterior resection (upper rectum)
  - Abdominoperineal resection and permanent sigmoid colostomy (lower rectum)
- Chemotherapy for patients with metastasis, residual disease, or recurrent inoperable tumor
- Radiation therapy (may be used before or after surgery or combined with chemotherapy) to induce tumor regression
- Referral to enterostomal therapist (if appropriate) for stoma management
- Nutritional support and guidelines
- Lifelong screening and testing for recurrence

Complex regional pain syndrome

- Chronic pain disorder resulting from abnormal healing after injury to a bone, muscle, or nerve
- Also known as reflex sympathetic dystrophy or causalgia

What causes it

- Cause unknown

Precipitating factors

- Trauma
- Herpes zoster infection
- Myocardial infarction
- Musculoskeletal disorder
- Malignancy

What to look for

- Aching throbbing and burning pain at site of injury, later may spread
- Altered blood flow to affected extremity
  – Change in limb temperature
  – Discoloration
  – Sweating
  – Swelling
- Skin, hair, and nail changes
- Muscle wasting and spasms
- Impaired mobility and weakness, contractures
- Osteoporosis

How it's treated

- Physical and occupational therapy to maintain function and independence
- Assistive devices as needed
- Anti-inflammatory drugs, vasodilators, and analgesics to treat symptoms
- Nerve or regional block for severe pain

Coronary artery disease

- Loss of oxygen and nutrients to heart tissue due to decreased coronary blood flow
- Can lead to acute coronary syndromes, such as unstable angina and acute myocardial infarction

What causes it

- Atherosclerosis (usual cause)
- Dissecting aneurysms, infectious vasculitis, syphilis, and congenital defects in the coronary vascular system
- Coronary artery spasms (Prinzmetal's angina)

Risk factors

- Family history of heart disease
- Age
- Hypertension
- Obesity
- Smoking
- Diabetes mellitus
- Stress
- Sedentary lifestyle
- High-fat, high-carbohydrate diet
- Abnormal serum lipid levels (total cholesterol, HDL, LDL, triglycerides)
- High blood homocysteine levels
- Menopause
- Infections producing inflammatory responses in the artery walls

What to look for

- Angina (primary symptom)
  - Burning, squeezing, or tightness in the substernal or precordial chest
  - May radiate to the left arm, neck, jaw, or shoulder blade

- – May follow physical exertion, emotional excitement, exposure to cold, or a large meal
- Nausea, vomiting, fainting, sweating, or cool extremities

Head of the class

Atypical chest pain in women

Women with coronary artery disease may experience typical chest pain (crushing chest pain that radiates down the arm or to the jaw), but they commonly experience atypical chest pain, vague chest pain, or a lack of chest pain.

Atypical symptoms include upper back discomfort between the shoulder blades, palpitations, a feeling of fullness in the neck, nausea, dizziness, unexplained fatigue, and exhaustion or shortness of breath.

How it's treated

- Nitrates to dilate coronary arteries and improve blood supply
- Beta-adrenergic blockers to decrease heart rate and lower the heart's oxygen demand
- Aspirin, glycoprotein IIb-IIIa inhibitors, and antithrombin drugs to reduce the risk of blood clots
- Calcium channel blockers to relax the coronary arteries and decrease afterload
- Angiotensin-converting enzyme inhibitors, diuretics, or other medications to lower blood pressure
- Antilipemics to treat abnormal lipid levels
- Percutaneous transluminal coronary angioplasty, rotational atherectomy, and stent placement to relieve occlusion
- Coronary artery bypass graft surgery
- Lifestyle modifications (dietary restrictions, smoking cessation, exercise, weight loss, stress reduction)

This is intense

Acute coronary syndrome

Acute occlusion of a coronary blood vessel and unstable angina are life-threatening emergencies. If your patient develops an acute coronary syndrome, expect to proceed as follows:

- Oxygen to increase oxygenation of blood
- Aspirin to inhibit platelet aggregation
- Nitroglycerin sublingually to relieve chest pain (unless systolic blood pressure is less than 90 mm Hg)
- Morphine to relieve pain
- Thrombolytic therapy (unless contraindicated) within 12 hours of onset of symptoms to restore vessel patency and minimize necrosis in ST-segment elevation MI
- I.V. heparin to promote patency in affected coronary artery
- Beta-adrenergic blockers to reduce myocardial workload
- Antiarrhythmic drugs, transcutaneous pacing patches (or transvenous pacemaker), defibrillation, or a combination of these methods to combat arrhythmias

- I.V. nitroglycerin for 24 to 48 hours (in patients without hypotension, bradycardia, or excessive tachycardia) to reduce afterload and preload and relieve chest pain
- Glycoprotein IIb/IIIa inhibitors (with non–ST-segment elevation MI with planned cardiac catheterization and positive troponin level) to reduce platelet aggregation
- Angiotensin-converting enzyme (ACE) inhibitors to reduce afterload and preload and prevent remodeling (begin in ST-segment elevation MI 6 hours after admission or when stable)
- PTCA to open blocked or narrowed arteries, or CABG if necessary.

Crohn's disease

- Slowly spreading, progressive inflammatory bowel disease
- Involves any part of GI tract, usually the proximal portion of the colon; also may affect the terminal ileum
- Extends through all layers of the intestinal wall

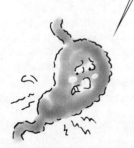

One of the characteristic signs of Crohn's disease is steady colicky pain in the right lower abdominal quadrant. Ouch, that hurts!

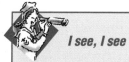

I see, I see

Bowel changes in Crohn's disease

As Crohn's disease progresses, fibrosis thickens the bowel wall and narrows the lumen. Narrowing (stenosis) can occur in any part of the intestine and cause varying degrees of intestinal obstruction. At first, the mucosa may appear normal, but as the disease progresses it takes on a "cobblestone" appearance, as shown.

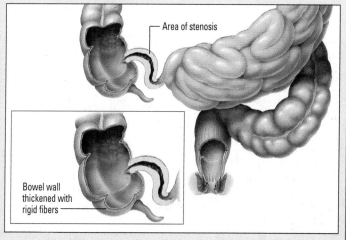

Area of stenosis

Bowel wall thickened with rigid fibers

What causes it

- Exact cause unknown
- Possibly results from immune reaction to virus or bacterium by causing ongoing intestinal inflammation

What to look for

- Protein-calorie malnutrition; nutrient deficiencies
- Dehydration

- Weight loss
- Diarrhea; steatorrhea (fatty stool)
- Intestinal obstruction
- Steady colicky pain in the right lower quadrant, cramping, tenderness
- Palpable mass in the right lower quadrant
- Bloody stool

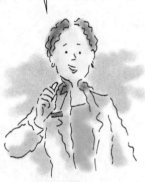

People with Crohn's disease often must take nutritional supplements to get the proper nutrients.

How it's treated

- Corticosteroids to reduce inflammation, diarrhea, pain, and bleeding
- Immunosuppressants to suppress response to antigens
- Sulfasalazine to reduce inflammation
- Infliximab to reduce inflammation
- Antidiarrheals to combat diarrhea (not used with significant bowel obstruction)
- Opioid analgesics to control pain and diarrhea
- Nutritional supplements to improve nutritional status
- Dietary modifications (elimination of foods that irritate mucosa or that stimulate excessive intestinal activity) to decrease bowel activity while still providing adequate nutrition
- Surgery to repair bowel perforation and correct massive hemorrhage, fistulas, or acute intestinal obstruction

Cushing's syndrome

- Cluster of clinical abnormalities caused by excessive corticotropin
- Cushing's disease (pituitary corticotropin excess) responsible for majority of endogenous cases

I see, I see

Understanding Cushing's syndrome

Prolonged exposure to pharmacologic doses of exogenous glucocorticoids	Secretory adrenocortical tumors stimulating adrenal cortex to increase corticotropin production

Excessive levels of glucocorticoids

Adrenal hyperplasia, suppression of pituitary corticotropin, and reduced hypothalamic secretion of corticotropin-releasing hormone

What causes it

- Excess of anterior pituitary hormone (corticotropin)
- Ectopic corticotropin secretion by tumor outside pituitary gland
- Excessive or prolonged use of glucocorticoids

What to look for

- Hallmark signs: rapidly developed adipose deposits on the face (moon face), neck, and trunk and purple striae on the skin
- Hypertension and fluid retention; heart failure
- Left ventricular hypertrophy
- Bleeding, petechiae, and ecchymosis
- Irritability and emotional lability; insomnia
- Diabetes mellitus
- Increased appetite and weight gain
- Peptic ulcers
- Susceptibility to infection and suppressed inflammatory response
- Muscle weakness, loss of muscle mass
- Pathologic fractures; skeletal growth retardation in children
- Increased sodium retention and potassium excretion
- Ureteral calculi
- Sexual dysfunction, mild virilism; acne and hirsutism in females
- Poor wound healing

How it's treated

- High-potassium, low-sodium, low-carbohydrate, low-calorie, high-protein diet to maintain nutritional balance
- Ketoconazole, metyrapone, and aminoglutethimide to inhibit cortisol synthesis
- Mitotane to destroy adrenocortical cells that secrete cortisol
- Bromocriptine and cyproheptadine to inhibit corticotropin secretion

- Surgical interventions (adrenalectomy, hypophysectomy, tumor resection) to control symptoms
- Radiation therapy to reduce or eliminate tumor, if present
- Control of hypertension, edema, diabetes, and cardiovascular symptoms
- Adequate rest and stress reduction

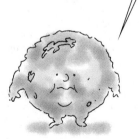

Treatment of Cushing's syndrome includes a combination of dietary changes, medication, rest, and possibly surgery or radiation to correct this hormonal imbalance.

Cystic fibrosis

- Chronic, progressive dysfunction of exocrine glands that affects multiple organ systems
- Most common fatal genetic disease in white children (typically of northern European descent)
- Carries average life expectancy of 32 years
- Characterized by chronic airway infection leading to bronchiectasis, bronchiolectasis, exocrine pancreatic insufficiency, intestinal dysfunction, abnormal sweat gland function, and reproductive dysfunction

I see, I see

Understanding cystic fibrosis

Cystic fibrosis typically arises from a mutation in the genetic coding of a single amino acid found in a protein called *cystic fibrosis transmembrane regulator* (CFTR). This protein, which is involved in the transport of chloride and other ions across cell membranes, resembles other transmembrane transport proteins but lacks phenylalanine (an essential amino acid) and, therefore, doesn't function properly.

Mutation in coding of amino acid

Interference with cAMP-regulated chloride channels and transport of other ions by preventing adenosine triphosphate from binding to the CFTR protein or by interfering with activation by protein kinase

Epithelial dysfunction in airways and intestines (volume-absorbing epithelia), sweat ducts (salt-absorbing epithelia), and pancreas (volume-secretory epithelia)

Dehydration, increased viscosity of mucus secretions, and obstruction of glandular ducts

What causes it

- Genetic mutation on chromosome 7q
- Possibly involves as many as 350 alleles within CFTR protein
- Transmitted by autosomal recessive inheritance

What to look for

- Obstructive lung changes (dry, nonproductive paroxysmal cough; dyspnea; tachypnea)
- Barrel chest
- Cyanosis and clubbing
- Crackles and wheezes
- Meconium ileus and jaundice in the neonate
- Poor growth and failure to thrive
- Frequent, bulky, foul-smelling, pale stool
- Ravenous appetite
- Distended abdomen, thin extremities
- Bowel obstruction
- Sallow skin with poor turgor
- Dehydration and fluid and electrolyte imbalances

How it's treated

- Hypertonic radiocontrast materials delivered by enema to treat acute obstructions due to meconium ileus
- Breathing exercises, postural drainage, and chest percussion to clear pulmonary secretions
- Antibiotics to treat lung infection (guided by sputum culture results)
- Bronchodilators and mucolytic agents to control airway constriction and increase mucus clearance
- Pancreatic enzyme replacement to maintain adequate nutrition
- Sodium-channel blockers to decrease sodium resorption from secretions and improve viscosity

- Uridine triphosphate to stimulate chloride secretion by non-CFTR proteins
- Sodium supplements to replace electrolytes lost through sweat
- Dornase alfa (genetically engineered pulmonary enzyme) to help liquefy mucus
- Recombinant alpha-antitrypsin to counteract excessive proteolytic activity produced during airway inflammation
- Gene therapy to introduce normal CFTR into affected epithelial cells
- Transplantation of heart or lungs for severe organ failure
- Referral for genetic counseling (Cystic Fibrosis Foundation) to discuss family planning issues or prenatal diagnosis options

Depression

- Major depression (unipolar disorder): syndrome of persistently sad mood lasting 2 weeks or longer
- May be a single episode or recurrent
- Can profoundly alter social, family, and occupational functioning
- Has suicide as its most serious consequence

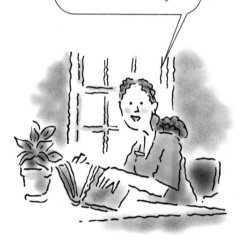

A person with clinical depression is typically persistently sad and has a cluster of other troubling symptoms that marks a change from his previous level of functioning.

What causes it
- Thought to be caused by abnormal levels of neurotransmitter chemicals in the brain that may be related to genetic, biological, and environmental factors
- Single stressful event can trigger episode in predisposed individual

Risk factors
- Gender (more common in females than in males)
- Advanced age
- Lower socioeconomic status
- Recent stressful experience, even positive ones like childbirth
- Chronic medical conditions and certain prescribed medications
- Underlying emotional or personality disorder
- Substance abuse
- Family history
- Lack of social support; recent loss of spouse
- Poor diet

What to look for
At least 5 of the following symptoms during the same 2-week period that are a change from previous functioning:
- Sad or "blue" feeling
- Loss of interest or pleasure in usual activities
- Significant weight loss or gain
- Insomnia or excessive sleeping
- Agitation or irritability
- Fatigue or loss of energy
- Feeling of worthlessness or excessive guilt
- Thoughts of death or suicide

This is intense

Recognizing suicide potential

A patient with a mood disorder may be at risk for attempting suicide. Stay alert for:
- overwhelming anxiety (the most frequent trigger for an attempt)
- withdrawal and social isolation
- saying farewell to friends and family
- putting affairs in order
- giving away prized possessions
- sending covert suicide messages and death wishes
- expressing obvious suicidal thoughts ("I'd be better off dead")
- describing a suicide plan
- hoarding medications
- talking about death and a feeling of futility
- behavior changes, especially as depression begins to subside.

Taking action

If you think your patient is at risk for suicide, take these steps:
- Keep the lines of communication open. Maintaining personal contact may help the suicidal patient feel he isn't alone or without resources or hope.
- To ensure a safe environment, check for dangerous conditions, such as exposed pipes, windows without safety glass, and access to the roof or open balconies.
- Remove belts, sharp objects such as razors, knives, nail files and clippers, suspenders, light cords, and glass from the patient's room.
- Make sure an acutely suicidal patient is observed around the clock. Stay alert when he uses a sharp object (as when shaving), takes medications, or uses the bathroom (to prevent hanging or other injury). Assign him a room near the nurses' station and with another patient.

How it's treated

- Selective serotonin reuptake inhibitors (SSRIs)—first-line antidepressant drugs
- Tricyclic antidepressants (TCAs)
- Monoamine oxidase (MAO) inhibitors for atypical depression or ineffective response to TCAs
- Electroconvulsive therapy (ECT) for severe or drug-resistant depression
- Supportive counseling for lifestyle and behavior changes
- Psychotherapy

Diabetes mellitus

- Chronic disorder of carbohydrate metabolism with subsequent alteration of protein and fat metabolism
- Characterized by hyperglycemia (elevated serum glucose level) resulting from lack of insulin, lack of insulin effect, or both
- General classifications
  - Type 1: absolute insulin insufficiency
  - Type 2: insulin resistance with varying degrees of insulin secretory defects
  - Pre-diabetes: blood glucose levels higher than normal but not high enough to be diagnosed with type 2 diabetes
  - Gestational (pregnancy-related) diabetes

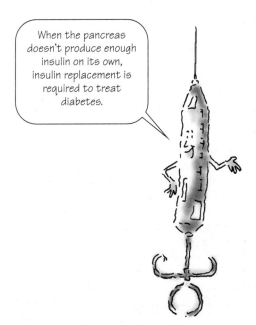

When the pancreas doesn't produce enough insulin on its own, insulin replacement is required to treat diabetes.

What causes it

Type 1 diabetes
- Autoimmune process triggered by viral or environmental factors
- Idiopathic (no evidence of autoimmune process)

Type 2 diabetes and pre-diabetes
- Beta cell exhaustion due to lifestyle habits or hereditary factors

Gestational diabetes
- Glucose intolerance, possibly a combination of insulin resistance and impaired insulin secretion, that occurs during pregnancy

Risk factors

Type 1 diabetes
- Autoimmune disorder (Addison's disease, celiac disease, thyroid autoimmunity, pernicious anemia)
- Family history
- Ethnicity (Black, Hispanic, Asian, or Native American)

Type 2 diabetes and pre-diabetes
- Obesity
- Family history
- Ethnicity (Black, Hispanic, Pacific Islander, Asian American, or Native American)
- History of gestational diabetes
- History of giving birth to an infant weighing more than 9 lb (4 kg)
- Hypertension
- Low high-density lipoprotein level (≤35 mg/dl)
- Elevated triglyceride level (≥250 mg/dl)
- Age older than 45 years

Gestational diabetes

- Pregnancy

What to look for

- Polyuria, polydipsia due to high serum osmolality (hyperglycemia)
- Polyphagia (occasionally in type 1 diabetes) from depleted cellular storage of carbohydrates, fats, and protein
- Weight loss from abnormal metabolism
- Headache, fatigue, lethargy from low intracellular glucose levels
- Muscle cramps, irritability, and emotional lability from electrolyte imbalances
- Vision changes from swelling
- Numbness and tingling from neural tissue damage
- Abdominal discomfort and pain; nausea, diarrhea, or constipation due to dehydration, electrolyte imbalances, or neuropathy
- Slow healing; skin itch; vaginal pruritus and vulvovaginitis due to hyperglycemia

How it's treated

Type 1 diabetes

- Insulin replacement (mixed-dose, split mixed-dose, or multiple daily injection regimens or continuous subcutaneous insulin infusions), meal planning, and exercise to normalize glucose levels and decrease complications
- Pancreas transplantation for poorly controlled diabetes to stabilize blood glucose levels and improve quality of life

Type 2 diabetes

- Oral antidiabetic drugs to stimulate endogenous insulin production, increase insulin sensitivity at the cellular level, suppress hepatic gluconeogenesis, and delay GI absorption of carbohydrates

- Insulin therapy (if uncontrolled with oral agents) to control blood glucose levels

Pre-diabetes

- Weight reduction of 5% to 10% of total body weight through diet and moderate exercise

Types 1 and 2 diabetes

- Careful monitoring of blood glucose levels to guide treatment
- Individualized meal plan to meet nutritional needs, control blood glucose and lipid levels, and maintain body weight
- Weight reduction (obese patient with type 2 diabetes mellitus) or high-calorie allotment, depending on growth stage and activity level (patient with type 1 diabetes mellitus) to ensure adequate nutrition
- Regular, daily physical exercise to help control glucose levels
- Patient and family education to inform about disease process, potential complications, nutritional management, exercise regimen, annual eye exams, daily inspection of feet, blood glucose self-monitoring, insulin, and oral medications

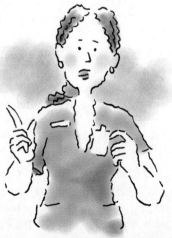

Obesity is a major risk factor for developing type 2 diabetes.

HHNS and DKA

Hyperosmolar hyperglycemic nonketotic syndrome (HHNS) and diabetic ketoacidosis (DKA) both are acute complications of diabetes. They share some similarities, but they are two distinct conditions. Treatment goals for both conditions include restoring fluid, electrolyte, and acid-base balance; controlling glucose levels; and providing cardiovascular and respiratory support in severe cases. Use the flowchart below to determine which condition your patient has.

Type 1 diabetes mellitus	Type 2 diabetes mellitus
YES	**YES**

Rapid onset	**NO**	Slow onset
YES		**YES**

• Drowsiness • Coma	• Extreme volume
• Stupor • Polyuria	depletion

YES

• Hyperventilation • Acetone breath odor • Blood glucose level slightly above normal • Mild hyponatremia • Positive or large serum ketone levels • Serum osmolality slightly elevated • Hyperkalemia initially, then hypokalemia • Metabolic acidosis	**NO**	• Slightly rapid respirations • No breath odor • Blood glucose level markedly elevated • Hypernatremia • Negative or small serum ketone levels • Serum osmolality markedly elevated • Normal serum potassium level • Lack of acidosis
YES		**YES**

Suspect DKA.	Suspect HHNS.

Gestational diabetes

- Nutrition therapy to control blood glucose levels
- Insulin (if diet alone is ineffective) to control blood glucose levels
- Postpartum counseling to address high risk of gestational diabetes in subsequent pregnancies and risk of type 2 diabetes later
- Regular exercise and prevention of weight gain to help prevent type 2 diabetes

Diverticular disease

- Characterized by bulging pouches (diverticula) in GI wall that push mucosal lining through surrounding muscle
- Classified by two clinical forms
  - Diverticulosis (when diverticula are present but don't cause symptoms)
  - Diverticulitis (when diverticula are inflamed, which may cause potentially fatal obstruction, infection, or hemorrhage)

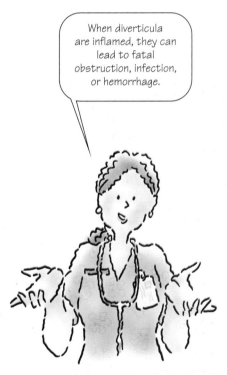

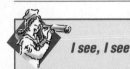

I see, I see

How diverticular disease develops

Diverticula probably result from high intraluminal pressure on an area of weakness in the GI wall where blood vessels enter.

In diverticular disease, retained undigested food and bacteria accumulate in the diverticular sac. This hard mass cuts off the blood supply to the thin walls of the sac, making the walls more susceptible to attack by colonic bacteria. Inflammation follows and may lead to perforation, abscess, peritonitis, obstruction, or hemorrhage.

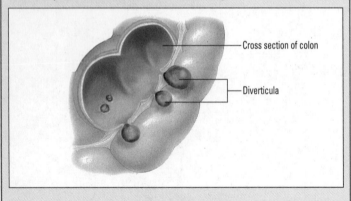

Cross section of colon

Diverticula

What causes it

- Diminished colonic motility and increased intraluminal pressure
- Low-fiber diet
- Defects in colon wall strength

What to look for

- Diverticulosis
  - Usually asymptomatic

  – May cause recurrent left lower quadrant pain accompanied by alternating constipation and diarrhea and relieved by defecation or passage of flatus
- Mild diverticulitis
  – Moderate left lower abdominal pain, mild nausea, gas, irregular bowel habits
  – Low-grade fever and leukocytosis
- Severe diverticulitis
  – Signs and symptoms of intestinal rupture, sepsis, and shock
  – Abdominal rigidity, left lower quadrant pain
  – High fever, chills, and hypotension
- Chronic diverticulitis
  – Ribbonlike stools and abdominal distention from fibrosis and adhesions causing incomplete obstruction
  – Diminishing or absent bowel sounds, nausea, vomiting, abdominal rigidity and pain if the obstruction increases

How it's treated

- Liquid or bland diet, stool softeners, and occasional doses of mineral oil to maintain bowel function
- High-residue diet (after pain has subsided) to help decrease intra-abdominal pressure during defecation
- Exercise to increase rate of stool passage
- Antibiotics to treat infection of diverticula
- Analgesics to control pain and relax smooth muscle
- Antispasmodics to control muscle spasms
- Colon resection with removal of involved segment in patients who don't respond to other treatment
- Temporary colostomy in diverticulitis accompanied by perforation, peritonitis, obstruction, or fistula to drain abscesses and rest colon
- Thorough patient education about fiber and other dietary habits to reduce recurrence

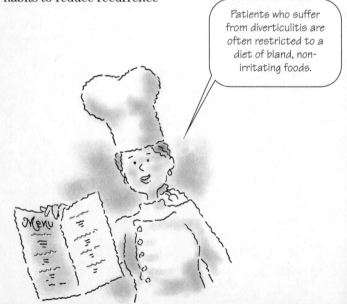

Patients who suffer from diverticulitis are often restricted to a diet of bland, non-irritating foods.

Emphysema

- Form of chronic obstructive pulmonary disease
- Characterized by abnormal, permanent enlargement of acini accompanied by destruction of alveolar walls
- Airflow limitation caused by lack of elastic recoil in lungs

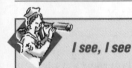

I see, I see

Understanding emphysema

In the patient with emphysema, recurrent pulmonary inflammation damages and eventually destroys the alveolar walls, creating large air spaces. The damaged alveoli can't recoil normally after expanding; therefore, bronchioles collapse.

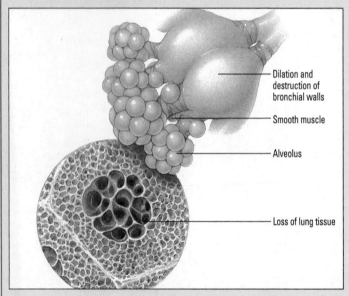

Dilation and destruction of bronchial walls

Smooth muscle

Alveolus

Loss of lung tissue

What causes it

- Cigarette smoking
- Alpha$_1$-antitrypsin deficiency

What to look for

- Tachypnea and dyspnea on exertion

- Barrel-shaped chest due to overinflation of the lungs
- Prolonged expiration and grunting due to use of accessory muscles
- Crackles, wheezing, decreased breath sounds
- Decreased chest expansion
- Hyperresonance of the chest on percussion
- Clubbed fingers and toes due to chronic hypoxia

How it's treated

- Avoidance of smoking and air pollution to preserve remaining alveoli
- Bronchodilators to reverse bronchospasm and promote mucociliary clearance
- Antibiotics to treat respiratory tract infections
- Pneumovax to prevent pneumococcal pneumonia
- Adequate hydration to liquefy and mobilize secretions
- Chest physiotherapy to mobilize secretions
- Oxygen therapy (low settings) to correct hypoxia
- Mucolytics to thin secretions and aid in mucus expectoration
- Aerosolized or systemic corticosteroids to decrease inflammation
- Alpha$_1$-antitrypsin replacement therapy, if appropriate
- Pulmonary rehabilitation program to teach breathing techniques, maximize exercise tolerance, and improve quality of life

Endometriosis

- Presence of endometrial tissue outside lining of uterine cavity (ectopic tissue)

What causes it

- Exact cause unknown
- May be related to:
  - retrograde menstruation with endometrial implantation at ectopic sites
  - genetic predisposition and depressed immune system
  - repeated inflammation inducing metaplasia of mesothelial cells to endometrial epithelium

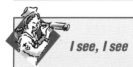

I see, I see

Understanding endometriosis

Ectopic endometrial tissue can implant almost anywhere in the peritoneum. It responds to normal stimulation in the same way as the endometrium, but more unpredictably. The endometrial cells respond to estrogen and progesterone with proliferation and secretion. During menstruation, the ectopic tissue bleeds, which causes inflammation of the surrounding tissues. This inflammation causes fibrosis, leading to adhesions that produce pain and infertility.

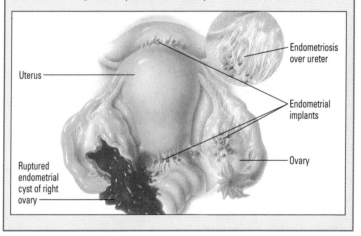

Uterus

Endometriosis over ureter

Endometrial implants

Ovary

Ruptured endometrial cyst of right ovary

What to look for

- Acquired dysmenorrhea—constant pain in the lower abdomen and vagina, posterior pelvis, and back that usually begins 5 to 7 days and lasts for 2 to 3 days after menses reaches its peak
- Other symptoms depending on location of ectopic tissue, including:
  – infertility

- profuse menses
- dyspareunia
- suprapubic pain, dysuria, and hematuria
- nausea and vomiting, which worsen before menses
- abdominal cramps
- pain on defecation, constipation, bloody stool

How it's treated

- Androgens, such as danazol, to slow growth of endometrial tissue outside uterus
- Progestins and continuous combined hormonal contraceptives (pseudopregnancy regimen) to relieve symptoms by causing regression of endometrial tissue
- Gonadotropin-releasing hormone agonists to induce pseudomenopause (medical oophorectomy), causing remission
- Mild analgesics or nonsteroidal anti-inflammatory agents for pain management
- Laparoscopic surgery (with conventional or laser techniques) to remove endometrial implants
- Presacral neurectomy for central pelvic pain
- Laparoscopic uterosacral nerve ablation for central pelvic pain
- Total abdominal hysterectomy (with or without bilateral salpingo-oophorectomy) as treatment of last resort for women who don't want to have children or for women who have extensive disease

Epilepsy

- Condition of the brain marked by susceptibility to recurrent seizures
- Also called seizure disorder
- Primary epilepsy: idiopathic without apparent brain changes
- Secondary epilepsy: characterized by structural or metabolic changes of the neuronal membrane

What causes it

- Idiopathic in about 50% of epilepsy cases
- Possible causes of secondary epilepsy
  - Anoxia after respiratory or cardiac arrest
  - Birth trauma: anoxia, blood incompatibility, or hemorrhage
  - Perinatal infection
  - Head injury or trauma
  - Infectious diseases, such as meningitis or encephalitis
  - Ingestion of toxins and substance abuse
  - Inherited or degenerative diseases
  - Metabolic disorders, such as hypoglycemia or hypoparathyroidism
  - Stroke
  - Brain tumors
  - Alcohol withdrawal (nonepileptic seizures)

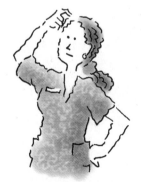

About half of all epilepsy cases have no known cause.

What to look for

- Generalized or grand mal seizures
  - Crying out, stiffening of body for a few seconds, followed by repetitive movement of arms and legs that often slows before completely stopping
  - Eyes usually open despite loss of consciousness
  - Apnea and cyanosis; deep breathing after the seizure
  - Urinary incontinence
  - Gradual return to consciousness (brief confusion may occur)
  - Drowsiness, fatigue, headache, muscle soreness, and limb weakness after the seizure
- Partial or focal seizure
  - Varying symptoms, depending on the part of the brain involved
  - Slow rhythmic movement or jerking of the affected part
  - Strange sensations
  - Small, repetitive movements such as picking at clothes or lip smacking
- Complex partial seizure
  - alterations in consciousness, such as amnesia and confusion
  - ability of patient to follow simple commands during the seizure
- Absence or petit mal seizures
  - Brief period (1 to 10 seconds) of impaired consciousness, evidenced by blinking or rolling of the eyes, a blank stare, and slight mouth movements
  - Can recur many times a day if not treated
  - May progress to a generalized seizure
- Status epilepticus
  - Continuous seizure state that can occur in all seizure types

This is intense

Status epilepticus

Status epilepticus is a life-threatening, continuous seizure state that may result from abrupt withdrawal of anticonvulsant medications, hypoxic or metabolic encephalopathy, acute head trauma, or septicemia due to encephalitis or meningitis. When treating a patient in this acute state, follow these guidelines:

- Establish and maintain the patient's airway.
- Administer oxygen and mechanical ventilation as appropriate.
- Administer fast-acting anticonvulsants such as diazepam or lorazepam I.V., as ordered.
- Administer longer acting anticonvulsants, such as phenytoin or fosphenytoin, as ordered.
- Be alert for respiratory depression and hypotension due to medications.
- Anticipate general anesthesia use if anticonvulsant therapy is ineffective.

- Monitor neurologic status frequently.
- Monitor vital signs and initiate continuous cardiac monitoring.
- Monitor blood glucose levels for hypoglycemia (a possible cause or effect of continuous seizures) and treat as ordered.
- Institute seizure precautions and ensure patient safety with raised, padded side rails, avoidance of restraints, and removal of dangerous objects.

How it's treated

- Anticonvulsants (such as phenytoin, carbamazepine, phenobarbital, or primidone) to treat generalized tonic-clonic seizures and complex partial seizures
- Valproic acid, clonazepam, and ethosuximide to treat absence seizures
- Routine monitoring of anticonvulsant medications
- Surgery to remove focal lesion if drug therapy fails

- Thiamine I.V. for chronic alcoholism or withdrawal
- Vagus nerve stimulator implant to reduce the incidence of partial seizures in drug-resistant cases
- Adequate sleep and stress management
- Alcohol avoidance

Fibromyalgia syndrome

- Diffuse chronic musculoskeletal pain syndrome
- Marked by 18 specific tender points
- May be primary disorder or associated with underlying disease, such as lupus, rheumatoid arthritis, osteoarthritis, sleep apnea syndrome, chronic fatigue syndrome, neck trauma, and HIV

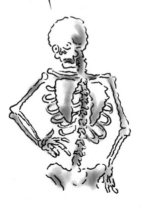

Tender points of fibromyalgia

The patient with fibromyalgia syndrome may complain of specific areas of tenderness, which are shown in the illustrations below.

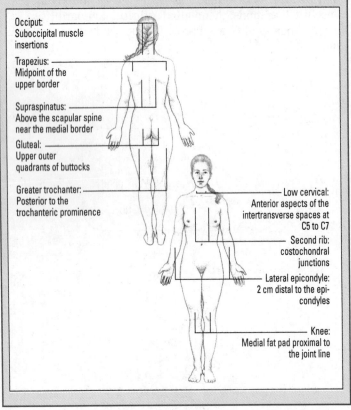

Occiput:
Suboccipital muscle insertions

Trapezius:
Midpoint of the upper border

Supraspinatus:
Above the scapular spine near the medial border

Gluteal:
Upper outer quadrants of buttocks

Greater trochanter:
Posterior to the trochanteric prominence

Low cervical:
Anterior aspects of the intertransverse spaces at C5 to C7

Second rib:
costochondral junctions

Lateral epicondyle:
2 cm distal to the epicondyles

Knee:
Medial fat pad proximal to the joint line

What causes it

- Unknown
- May be multifactorial and influenced by physical and mental stress, physical conditioning, and quality of sleep
- May have neuroendocrine, psychiatric, and hormonal factors or relationship to infection

What to look for

- Diffuse, dull, aching pain typically concentrated across the neck, shoulders, lower back, and proximal limbs
- Worse in the morning and may be accompanied by stiffness
- Varying level of pain each day, exacerbated by stress, lack of sleep, weather changes, and inactivity
- Irritable bowel syndrome
- Tension headaches
- "Puffy hands" (sensation of hand swelling, especially in the morning)
- Paresthesia
- Painful menstrual periods
- "Foggy" thinking and memory

How it's treated

- Low-impact aerobic exercise to improve conditioning, energy levels, and sense of well-being
- Well-balanced diet and avoidance of caffeine
- Steroids or lidocaine, massage therapy, and ultrasound treatments for problematic areas
- Acupuncture, phototherapy, yoga, and tai chi
- Tricyclic antidepressants at bedtime to aid sleep
- Serotonin reuptake inhibitor to relieve symptoms

Gastroesophageal reflux disease (GERD)

- Backflow of gastric or duodenal contents (or both) into the esophagus and past the lower esophageal sphincter (LES) without associated belching or vomiting
- Reflux of gastric contents that causes acute epigastric pain, usually after meals

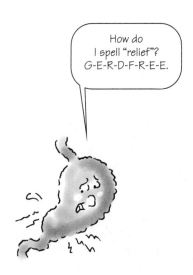

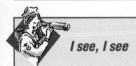

I see, I see

How GERD develops

Hormonal fluctuations, mechanical stress, and the effects of certain foods and drugs can decrease LES pressure. When LES pressure falls and intra-abdominal or intragastric pressure rises, the normally contracted LES relaxes inappropriately and allows reflux of gastric acid or bile secretions into the lower esophagus. There, the reflux irritates and inflames the esophageal mucosa, causing pyrosis (heartburn).

Persistent inflammation can cause LES pressure to decrease further, possibly triggering a recurrent cycle of reflux and pyrosis.

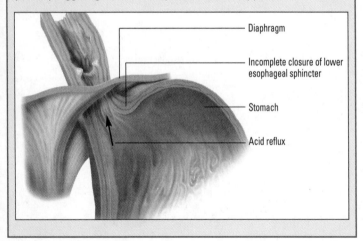

- Diaphragm
- Incomplete closure of lower esophageal sphincter
- Stomach
- Acid reflux

What causes it

- Weakened esophageal sphincter
- Increased abdominal pressure (obesity, pregnancy)
- Hiatal hernia
- Medications (morphine, diazepam, calcium channel blockers, meperidine, anticholinergic agents)

- Alcohol, cigarettes, and foods that lower LES pressure
- Nasogastric intubation for more than 4 days
- Increased gastric secretions from physiological and psychological stress

What to look for

- Heartburn
  - May become more severe with vigorous exercise, bending, or lying down and following a meal
  - May be relieved by antacids or sitting upright
- Chronic pain that mimics angina pectoris, with radiation to the neck, jaws, and arms; results from esophageal spasms
- Painful swallowing, dysphagia due to reflux
- Halitosis
- Bloody vomitus
- Nocturnal regurgitation
- Chronic cough, hoarseness, or nocturnal wheezing from throat irritation
- Weight loss
- Signs of aspiration, such as dyspnea and recurrent lung infection

How it's treated

- Diet modification (frequent, small meals; avoidance of eating before bedtime) to reduce abdominal pressure and decrease incidence of reflux
- Low-fat, high-fiber diet and avoidance of caffeine, alcohol, and carbonated beverages to decrease gastric acid stimulation
- Positioning (sitting up during and after meals; sleeping with the head of the bed elevated) to reduce abdominal pressure and prevent reflux
- Increased fluid intake to wash gastric contents out of the esophagus
- Antacids to neutralize acidic content and minimize irritation
- Cytoprotective agents to minimize mucosal damage
- Histamine-2 receptor antagonists to inhibit gastric acid secretion
- Proton pump inhibitors to reduce gastric acidity
- Cholinergic agents to increase LES pressure
- Smoking cessation or weight loss to increase LES pressure
- Surgery to repair hiatal hernia, if appropriate

Glaucoma

- Abnormally high intraocular pressure (IOP), which can damage the optic nerve
- Results from either overproduction or obstruction of the outflow of aqueous humor
- Can lead to gradual, permanent peripheral vision loss and blindness if left untreated

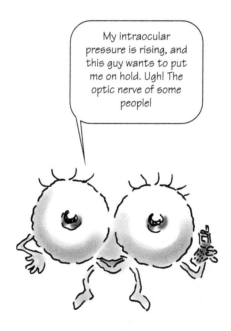

What causes it

- Chronic open-angle glaucoma—familial; associated with diabetes and hypertension
- Acute angle-closure (narrow-angle) glaucoma—more common in African Americans, in those with a family history of glaucoma, and in those who use systemic anticholinergics, such as atropine or eye dilation drops
- Secondary glaucoma—results from infection, trauma, ocular neoplasm, or medications, such as steroids
- Congenital glaucoma—occurs due to scarring from infections or retinopathy of prematurity

What to look for

- Chronic open-angle glaucoma
  - Bilateral with insidious onset; symptoms appear late in disease
  - Halos around lights
  - Loss of peripheral vision
  - Mild aching in eyes
  - Reduced visual acuity, especially at night, that's not correctable
- Acute angle-closure glaucoma
  - Rapid onset, usually unilateral
  - Acute pain in inflamed eye; pressure over the eye
  - Blurring and decreased visual acuity
  - Halos around lights
  - Cloudy cornea
  - Moderate pupil dilation that's nonreactive to light
  - Photophobia
- Nausea and vomiting from increased IOP

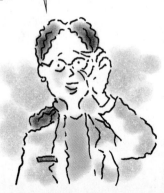

Be on the lookout for the signs of glaucoma to prevent permanent vision loss.

How it's treated

- Miotic eye drops, such as pilocarpine, epinephrine, or dipivefrin, to improve outflow of aqueous humor
- Beta-blocker eye drops, such as timolol or betaxolol, to decrease aqueous humor production
- Alpha$_2$-adrenoreceptor agonist eye drops, such as brimonidine, a longer acting medication that decreases production of and increases outflow of aqueous humor
- Prostaglandin eye drops, such as latanoprost, to increase outflow
- Carbonic anhydrase inhibitors to decrease aqueous humor production
- Laser surgery to increase outflow if unresponsive to drug therapy
- Trabeculectomy to improve aqueous outflow
- Aqueous shunt to drain excess fluid
- Cytophotocoagulation laser therapy to decrease aqueous humor production

Gout

- Metabolic disease in which urate deposits cause painfully arthritic joints
- Characterized by overproduction of uric acid, retention of uric acid, or both
- Can affect any joint but occurs most often in the feet and legs
- Can be a primary disease or secondary to other disorders

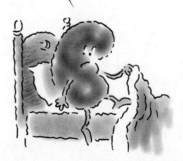

Gout results when uric acid crystals accumulate in joints, causing pain and inflammation, often in the feet and legs. Bed rest can help relieve acute flare-ups.

What causes it

- Primary gout—unknown; may be a genetic defect
- Secondary gout—associated with alcohol use, obesity, diabetes mellitus, hypertension, hyperlipidemia, and renal disease; drug therapy with aspirin, hydrochlorothiazide, or pyrazinamide; and increased cell death due to chemotherapy

What to look for

- Intermittent episodes of joint pain, lasting for days or weeks
- Hot, inflamed, dusky red, or cyanotic joints
- Low-grade fever
- Chronic changes, including persistent, painful polyarthritis, with large, subcutaneous tophi
- Ulcerated skin over the tophus, with chalky, white exudate or pus
- Chronic renal dysfunction
- Hypertension
- Albuminuria and urolithiasis

How it's treated

- Bed rest, immobilization, and protection of affected joints
- Local application of heat or cold for acute attacks
- Analgesic and nonsteroidal anti-inflammatory drugs
- Steroid drugs or joint injections in severe cases
- Colchicine to decrease deposits and reduce inflammation
- Chronic allopurinol use to suppress uric acid formation and prevent further attacks
- Uricosuric agents, such as probenecid and sulfinpyrazone, to promote uric acid excretion in patients with normal renal function
- Dietary modification to reduce purine intake from anchovies, organ meats, lentils, asparagus, mushrooms, and sardines
- Avoidance of alcohol, which raises urate level
- Adequate fluid intake
- Gradual weight loss
- Surgery in severe cases to improve joint function or drain infected or ulcerated tophi

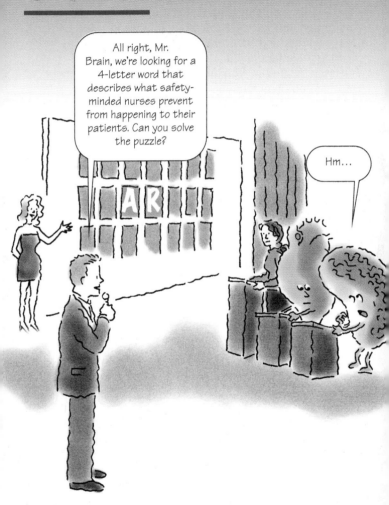

Headache, migraine

- Throbbing, vascular headache that usually first appears in childhood and recurs throughout adulthood
- May be classified according to presence of aura
  – common migraine: no aura (80% of cases)
  – classic migraine: with aura (20% of cases)
- More common in women; strong familial incidence

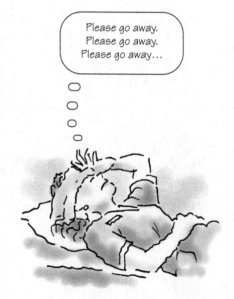

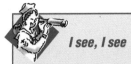

I see, I see

How migraine headache develops

Migraine headaches are thought to be associated with constriction and dilation of intracranial and extracranial arteries. Neurogenic inflammation can cause local vasoconstriction of innervated cerebral arteries and reduced cerebral blood flow. Compensatory vasodilation and biochemical abnormalities, including local leakage of neurokinin through dilated arteries and decreased plasma level of serotonin, result.

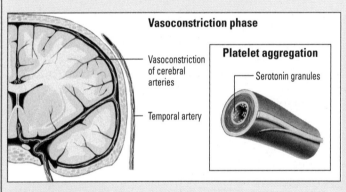

Vasoconstriction phase

Vasoconstriction of cerebral arteries

Temporal artery

Platelet aggregation

Serotonin granules

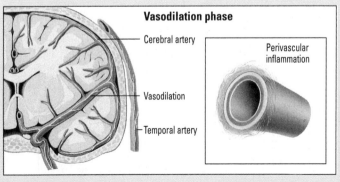

Vasodilation phase

Cerebral artery

Vasodilation

Temporal artery

Perivascular inflammation

What causes it

- Exact cause unknown
- Possible triggering mechanism: dysfunction of trigeminal nerve pathway
- Contributing factors
  - Change in routine (sleep, missed meals)
  - Caffeine intake
  - Change in hormone levels (women)
  - Emotional stress or fatigue
  - Environmental stimuli (noise, crowds, bright lights, weather)

What to look for

- Unilateral pulsating pain, which may become generalized
- Reports of preceding aura: scintillating scotoma (zig-zag lines), hemianopia, unilateral paresthesia, speech impairment
- Irritability, anorexia, nausea, vomiting, and photophobia

How it's treated

- Abortive medications (serotonin $5HT_1$-receptor agonists, dihydroergotamine, nonsteroidal anti-inflam-

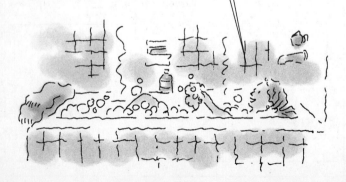

Too much stress can bring on a migraine. I have to remember to take some time for myself!

matory drugs) to relieve pain (early treatment of symptoms is most effective)

- Antiemetic drugs to treat nausea and vomiting
- Biofeedback and massage to relieve or reduce pain
- Beta-adrenergic blockers, clonidine, or amitriptyline to prevent migraine attacks
- Avoidance of contributing factors to prevent migraine attacks
- Maintenance of headache diary to help determine headache triggers

Heart failure

- Syndrome that occurs when heart can't pump enough blood to meet body's metabolic needs
- Results in intravascular and interstitial volume overload and poor tissue perfusion
- May be classified according to side of heart affected (left- or right-sided heart failure) or cardiac cycle involved (systolic or diastolic dysfunction)

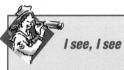

I see, I see

Understanding heart failure

Left-sided heart failure	Right-sided heart failure
Ineffective left ventricular contractility	Ineffective right ventricular contractility
Reduced left ventricular pumping ability	Reduced right ventricular pumping ability
Decreased cardiac output to body	Decreased cardiac output to lungs
Blood backup into left atrium and lungs	Blood backup into right atrium and peripheral circulation
Pulmonary congestion, dyspnea, activity intolerance	Weight gain, peripheral edema, engorgement of kidneys, liver, and other organs
Pulmonary edema and right-sided heart failure	

What causes it

- Abnormal cardiac muscle function
- Abnormal left ventricular volume, pressure, or filling

Risk factors

- Heart diseases (such as rheumatoid, atherosclerotic, congenital)
- Hypertension
- Cardiomyopathy
- Valvular disease

- Arrhythmias
- Pregnancy and childbirth
- Thyrotoxicosis
- Pulmonary embolism
- COPD
- Severe infection

What to look for

- Dyspnea, orthopnea, paroxysmal nocturnal dyspnea, hypoxia, nonproductive cough and crackles due to pulmonary congestion
- Fatigue
- Displacement of the point of maximal impulse (PMI) toward the left axillary line
- Tachycardia, palpitations, arrhythmias
- Hypertension
- Ventricular gallop
- Cool, pale skin
- Jugular vein distention, liver engorgement, positive hepatojugular reflux and right upper quadrant pain due to venous congestion
- Anorexia, fullness, and nausea due to organ congestion
- Nocturia
- Weight gain and edema, ascites, or anasarca due to fluid excess

This is intense

Managing pulmonary edema

If your patient's heart failure progresses to pulmonary edema, follow these guidelines:
• Provide oxygen and anticipate endotracheal intubation and mechanical ventilation.
• Monitor arterial blood gas levels, vital signs, oxygen saturation, breath sounds, intake and output, and pulmonary artery catheter pressures.
• Begin continuous cardiac monitoring and treat arrhythmias.
• Administer diuretics to mobilize fluids.
• Administer positive inotropic agents, such as digoxin and inamrinone, to enhance contractility.
• Administer vasopressors to enhance contractility and promote systemic vasoconstriction for hypotension.
• Administer vasodilators, such as nitroprusside, to decrease peripheral vascular resistance, preload, and afterload.
• Give morphine to reduce anxiety and dyspnea and to dilate the systemic venous bed. Monitor for respiratory depression.
• Provide emotional support and explain all procedures.

How it's treated

• ACE inhibitors or vasodilators to reduce peripheral vascular resistance and afterload
• Digoxin to increase myocardial contractility, thereby improving cardiac output and regulating rhythm
• Diuretics to reduce fluid volume overload and venous return
• Beta-adrenergic blockers in patient with New York Heart Association (NYHA) class II or III heart failure caused by left ventricular systolic dysfunction to prevent remodeling and to regulate rhythm

- Carvedilol, a nonselective beta-adrenergic blocker with alpha-receptor blockade, to decrease afterload in addition to beta-blocker effects
- Inotropic therapy with dopamine, dobutamine, or milrinone for acute treatment of heart failure
- Lifestyle modifications (exercise; weight loss; reduced sodium, alcohol, and fat intake; smoking cessation; stress reduction) to reduce symptoms of heart failure
- Valve replacement surgery for heart failure due to valve dysfunction
- CABG surgery or angioplasty for heart failure due to coronary artery disease
- Biventricular pacemaker in patient with NYHA class III or IV heart failure to reduce symptoms and improve quality of life
- Heart transplantation for patient receiving aggressive medical treatment but still experiencing limitations or repeated hospitalizations

Hemochromatosis

- Inherited disorder in which too much iron is absorbed and stored by the body
- Organ damage leading to cirrhosis, diabetes, cardiomegaly with heart failure and arrhythmias

What causes it

- Autosomal recessive genetic defect
- Causes of juvenile and neonatal types unclear

What to look for

- Joint pain
- Fatigue
- Weight loss
- Abdominal pain
- Decreased libido
- Bronze or gray-colored skin
- Signs and symptoms of other disorders, such as liver disease or cancer, diabetes, arthritis, and heart failure

How it's treated

- Phlebotomy to remove excess iron
- Dietary modifications to avoid iron-rich foods, alcohol, and iron and vitamin C supplements
- Supportive care for pain and secondary disorders
- Genetic counseling for family members

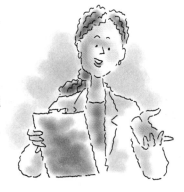

Too much iron circulating in the body can lead to hemochromatosis.

Hemophilia

- X-linked-inherited recessive bleeding disorder that results in deficiency or absence of clotting factors
- Varying severity and prognosis, depending on degree of deficiency and site of bleeding
- Classification depends on clotting factor involved
  - Hemophilia A (classic hemophilia)—deficiency of clotting factor VIII; affects more than 80% of those with hemophilia
  - Hemophilia B—results from deficiency of factor IX; affects 15% of those with disorder
- Prevention of crippling deformities and prolonged life expectancy possible with proper treatment

I see, I see

Understanding hemophilia

Deficiency in factor VIII (hemophilia A) or factor IX (hemophilia B)

▼

Inability to activate factor X (key enzyme that controls conversion of fibrinogen to fibrin)

▼

Inability to form a stable fibrin clot

▼

Excessive bleeding when clotting factors are reduced by more than 75%

What causes it

- Chromosomal defect
  - Specific gene on X chromosome that codes for factor VIII synthesis (hemophilia A)
  - Substitution of more than 300 different base-pair genes on X chromosome that code for factor IX (hemophilia B)

What to look for

- Spontaneous bleeding in severe hemophilia
- Excessive or continued bleeding or bruising after minor trauma or surgery
- Large subcutaneous and deep intramuscular hematomas with mild traumas
- Prolonged bleeding with mild hemophilia after major trauma or surgery
- Pain, swelling, and tenderness from bleeding into joints, especially weight-bearing joints
- Internal bleeding, commonly seen as abdominal, chest, or flank pain
- Hematuria
- Hematemesis or tarry stool

How it's treated

- Clotting factor replacement therapy to prevent or treat bleeding episodes
- Antifibrolytic drugs, such as aminocaproic acid and tranexamic acid, to inhibit clot breakdown during oral bleeding episodes and mild intestinal bleeding
- Prophylactic desmopressin before dental procedures or minor surgery to release stored von Willebrand's factor and factor VIII, thereby reducing bleeding
- Use of clothing with padded patches on knees and elbows (young children) to prevent injury that could lead to bleeding

- Avoiding contact sports (older children) to prevent injury that could lead to bleeding
- Referral of patients and carriers for genetic counseling to discuss family planning issues

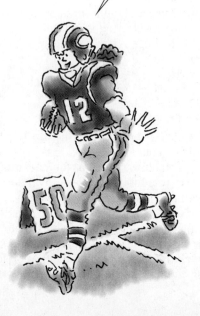

Children with hemophilia should avoid participating in contact sports, which can cause injuries that lead to bleeding.

Hepatitis B

- Common liver infection that causes hepatic cell destruction, necrosis, and autolysis
- Spread through contact with contaminated blood, secretions, and stool
- Type D hepatitis: linked to chronic hepatitis B infection
- Chronic hepatitis B: diagnosed when HBsAg test is positive for at least 6 months

What causes it

- Infection with causative virus

What to look for

- May be asymptomatic
- Flulike symptoms: fatigue, fever
- Enlarged liver and spleen
- Ascites and pedal edema
- Jaundice
- Dark-colored urine and pale stools
- Cirrhosis
  - Abdominal pain
  - Diarrhea or constipation
  - Nausea and vomiting
  - Muscle cramps
  - Chronic dyspepsia
  - Pruritus
  - Weight loss
  - Bleeding tendencies

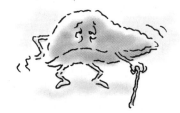

How it's treated

- Interferon alpha, adefovir dipivoxil, lamivudine, or entecavir for virus control
- Rest to minimize energy demands
- Avoidance of alcohol and drugs to prevent further hepatic damage
- Diet modification (small, high-calorie meals) to combat anorexia
- Supplemental vitamins and feedings to improve nutritional status
- Parenteral nutrition (if patient can't eat because of persistent vomiting) to maintain adequate nutritional status
- Vaccination against hepatitis A to provide immunity before transmission occurs and to prevent possible further damage
- Blood-borne and enteric precautions to prevent spread of infection
- Supportive treatment of cirrhosis, such as antiemetics, paracentesis, fluid and sodium restriction, and diuretics

Hepatitis C

- Common liver infection that causes hepatic cell destruction, necrosis, and autolysis
- Blood-borne disease associated with shared needles, blood transfusions, and sexual transmission
- Diagnosed when antibodies to anti-hepatitis C are present and serum aminotransferase levels remain elevated for more than 6 months

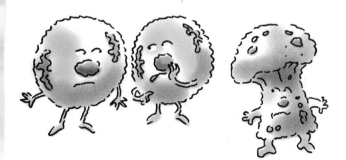

What causes it
- Infection with causative virus

What to look for
- May be asymptomatic
- Flulike symptoms: fatigue, fever
- Enlarged liver and spleen
- Ascites and pedal edema
- Jaundice
- Dark-colored urine and pale stools
- Cirrhosis
  - Abdominal pain
  - Diarrhea or constipation
  - Nausea and vomiting
  - Muscle cramps
  - Chronic dyspepsia
  - Pruritus
  - Weight loss
  - Bleeding tendencies

How it's treated
- Antivirals interferon alpha and pegylated interferon in combination with ribavirin
- Rest to minimize energy demands
- Avoidance of alcohol and drugs to prevent further hepatic damage
- Diet modification (small, high-calorie meals) to combat anorexia
- Supplemental vitamins and feedings to improve nutritional status
- Parenteral nutrition (if patient can't eat because of persistent vomiting) to maintain adequate nutritional status
- Vaccination against hepatitis A and B to provide immunity before transmission occurs and to prevent possible further damage

- Standard precautions to prevent spread of infection
- Supportive treatment of cirrhosis, such as antiemetics, paracentesis, fluid and sodium restriction, and diuretics

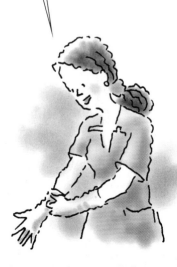

Herpes simplex type 2

- Recurrent viral infection caused by *Herpesvirus hominis*
- Characterized by painful, fluid-filled vesicles that appear in genital area (some cases remain subclinical with no symptoms)
- Largely supportive treatment; no known cure
- Also known as genital herpes

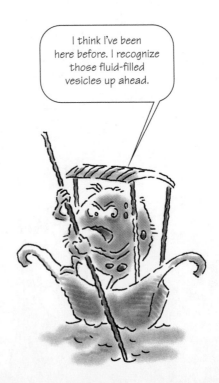

I think I've been here before. I recognize those fluid-filled vesicles up ahead.

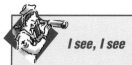

I see, I see

Understanding herpes simplex type 2

Herpes simplex type 2 is transmitted by contact with infectious lesions or secretions. The virus infiltrates the skin, local replication of the virus occurs, and the virus enters cutaneous neurons. After the patient becomes infected, a latency period follows, although repeated outbreaks may develop at any time.

Initial infection
Highly infectious period, with symptoms appearing after incubation period (average period: 1 week)

Latency
Intermittently infectious period, marked by viral dormancy or viral shedding and no disease symptoms

Recurrent infection
Highly infectious period similar to initial infection, with milder symptoms that resolve faster

What causes it

- Transmission of *Herpesvirus hominis* (causes type 1 and type 2 herpes)
  - Primarily by sexual contact
  - Possibly by autoinoculation with type 1 herpes (through poor hand-washing practices or orogenital sex)
- Pregnancy-related transmission
  - Transmission of virus possible from infected pregnant patient to neonate during vaginal delivery
  - Cesarean delivery recommended during initial infection when active lesions are present

What to look for
- Reports of tingling or itching in the genital area
- Pain in the buttocks or down the leg
- Fluid-filled vesicles that ulcerate and heal in 1 to 3 weeks
- Fever
- Regional lymphadenopathy
- Recurrent outbreaks that are usually mild and brief

How it's treated
- Suppressive or episodic therapy with antiviral drugs (acyclovir, valacyclovir, famciclovir) to decrease severity and shorten duration of lesions, decrease viral shedding, and decrease frequency of recurrence
- Analgesics and antipyretics to reduce fever and relieve pain
- Warm baths, cool compresses, or topical anesthetics to help reduce pain
- Education and counseling to provide patient with information about care measures during outbreaks, prevention of secondary or recurrent herpes infections (including eye infections), measures to avoid infecting others (avoiding sexual activity during active stage, using condoms), and risks of fetal infection

Human immunodeficiency virus (HIV) infection

- Gradual destruction of cell-mediated (T cell) immunity and autoimmunity, causing susceptibility to opportunistic infections, cancer, and other abnormalities
- Acquired immunodeficiency syndrome (AIDS) caused by blood or body-fluid transmission of HIV
- Diagnosis of AIDS based on HIV status and presence of fewer than 200 CD4+ T cells per cubic millimeter of blood

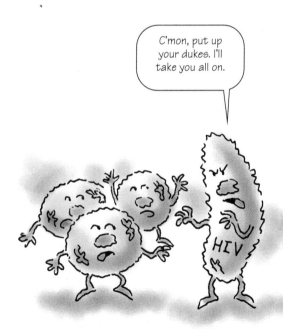

I see, I see

Understanding AIDS

HIV retrovirus enters body and strikes helper T cells bearing the CD4⁻ antigen.

▼

HIV copies its genetic material in reverse manner, allowing for production of DNA from its viral RNA.

▼

Viral DNA enters cell's nucleus, where it becomes incorporated with host cell's DNA and transcribed into more viral RNA.

▼

Host cell reproduces, duplicating its viral DNA and passing it on to its newly formed daughter cells.

▼

Viral enzymes (proteases) arrange RNA into viral particles.

▼

Viral particles move to periphery of host cell, where viral buds emerge and travel to infect other cells.

▼

HIV infection destroys CD4⁺ cells, other immune cells, and neuroglial cells.

What causes it

- Contact with HIV-infected blood or other body fluids (HIV-1 or HIV-2)

Risk factors

- Sharing drug needles or syringes
- Sexual contact with HIV-infected person (whether diagnosed or not) without use of a barrier (such as a condom)
- Prenatal exposure

What to look for
- May be asymptomatic for months or years
- Nonspecific symptoms (generalized adenopathy, weight loss, fatigue, night sweats, fever)
- Neurologic dysfunction (AIDS dementia complex, HIV encephalopathy, and peripheral neuropathies)
- Immunodeficiency (opportunistic infections and unusual cancers)
- Autoimmunity (lymphoid interstitial pneumonitis, arthritis, hypergammaglobulinemia, and production of autoimmune antibodies)

How it's treated
- Primary therapy—combination of three different antiretroviral agents to inhibit HIV replication with fewest adverse reactions
- Current recommendations—use of two nucleosides (which interfere with copying of viral RNA into DNA by reverse transcriptase) plus one protease inhibitor (to block replication of virus particle and reduce number of new virus particles produced), or two nucleosides and one non-nucleoside (which interfere with action of reverse transcriptase) to inhibit production of resistant, mutant strains
- Immunomodulatory agents to boost immune system weakened by AIDS and retroviral therapy
- Human granulocyte colony-stimulating growth factor to stimulate neutrophil production (retroviral therapy causes anemia, so patients may receive epoetin alfa)
- Anti-infective and antineoplastic agents to combat opportunistic infections and associated cancers (some prophylactically to help resist opportunistic infections)
- Immunizations against pneumonia and influenza
- Supportive therapy (nutritional support, fluid and electrolyte replacement therapy, pain relief, psychological support) to provide comfort

- Diligent practice of standard precautions to prevent inadvertent transmission of AIDS and other infectious diseases transmitted by similar routes
- Information about AIDS societies and support programs to educate and support patient and significant other

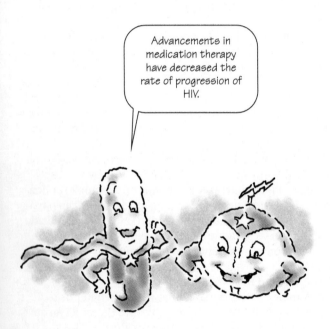

Huntington's disease

- Hereditary disease in which degeneration of the cerebral cortex and basal ganglia causes chronic progressive chorea and mental deterioration and dementia
- Also known as Huntington's chorea

What causes it

- Autosomal dominant genetic trait

What to look for

- Insidious onset, usually between ages 35 and 55
- Loss of musculoskeletal control and development of progressively severe choreic movements—rapid, violent, and purposeless
- Balance and coordination difficulties
- Difficulty shifting gaze without moving head
- Hesitant, halting, or slurred speech
- Difficulty swallowing
- Personality changes
  - Obstinence
  - Carelessness and apathy
  - Untidiness
  - Moodiness
  - Inappropriate behavior
  - Loss of memory and concentration
- Progressive dementia

How it's treated

- No known cure—treatment is supportive, protective, and symptomatic
- Dopamine blockers, tranquilizers, and antipsychotic drugs to help control choreic movements and reduce abnormal behaviors
- Antidepressants to treat associated depression and mood swings

- Reserpine, tetrabenazine, and amantadine to control extra movements
- Coenzyme Q10 to decrease disease progression
- Speech, physical, and occupational therapy to address safety issues and promote functioning as long as possible
- Genetic counseling for family members, as appropriate

Hypertension

- Intermittent or sustained elevation of blood pressure
- Occurs as two major types: essential (primary or idiopathic) hypertension and secondary hypertension
- Major cause of stroke, cardiac disease, and renal failure

I see, I see

Understanding hypertension

To understand hypertension, you must first understand that arterial blood pressure is a product of cardiac output (CO) and total peripheral resistance (TPR). CO is increased by conditions that increase heart rate, stroke volume, or both. TPR is increased by factors that increase blood viscosity or reduce the lumen size of vessels, especially the arterioles.

Several theories help explain how hypertension develops, including:
• changes in the arteriolar bed, causing increased TPR
• abnormally increased tone in the sympathetic nervous system, causing increased TPR
• increased blood volume resulting from renal or hormonal dysfunction
• increased arteriolar thickening caused by genetic factors, leading to increased TPR
• abnormal renin release, resulting in formation of angiotensin II, which constricts the arteriole and increases blood volume.

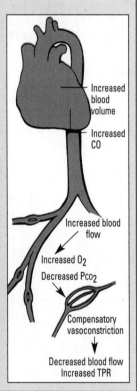

Increased blood volume

Increased CO

Increased blood flow

Increased O_2
Decreased Pco_2

Compensatory vasoconstriction

Decreased blood flow
Increased TPR

What causes it

Primary hypertension
• Unknown

Secondary hypertension
• Renal artery stenosis and parenchymal disease

- Brain tumor, quadriplegia, and head injury
- Pheochromocytoma, Cushing's syndrome, hyperaldosteronism, and thyroid, pituitary, or parathyroid dysfunction
- Hormonal contraceptives, cocaine, epoetin alfa, sympathetic stimulants, monoamine oxidase inhibitors taken with tyramine, estrogen replacement therapy, and nonsteroidal anti-inflammatory drugs (NSAIDs)

Risk factors

Primary hypertension
- Diabetes mellitus
- Family history, advancing age
- Obesity, sedentary lifestyle
- Stress
- Tobacco use; high intake of sodium, saturated fat, alcohol

What to look for
- Elevated blood pressure
  - Greater than 139 mm Hg systolic, or 89 mm Hg diastolic reading on at least 2 consecutive occasions
  - Readings of 120 to 139 mm Hg systolic, or 80 to 89 mm Hg diastolic in pre-hypertension
- Occipital headache; may worsen in the morning
- Nausea and vomiting
- Epistaxis
- Dizziness, confusion, blurred vision
- Nocturia
- Edema
- Fatigue

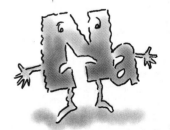

Hypertension can be controlled by reducing sodium intake.

- Bruits over the abdominal aorta, carotid, renal or femoral arteries due to stenosis or aneurysm

How it's treated

- Lifestyle modifications (exercise; weight loss; reduced sodium, alcohol, and fat intake; smoking cessation; stress reduction) to reduce symptoms
- Drug therapy (thiazide-type diuretic, ACE inhibitor, angiotensin receptor blocker, beta-adrenergic blocker, calcium channel blocker, or combination) to treat primary hypertension
- Correction of underlying cause and control of hypertensive effects to treat secondary hypertension

Hyperthyroidism

- Metabolic imbalance that results from overproduction of thyroid hormone; also called thyrotoxicosis
- In Graves' disease (most common form), increased thyroxine (T4) production causes enlarged thyroid gland (goiter) and multiple system changes

I see, I see

Understanding hyperthyroidism

T-cell lymphocytes become sensitized to thyroid antigens and stimulate B-cell lymphocytes to secrete autoantibodies.

▼

Thyroid-stimulating antibodies bind to and stimulate thyroid-stimulating hormone (TSH) receptors of the thyroid gland.

▼

This stimulation increases production of thyroid hormone and cell growth.

What causes it

- Autoimmune disease (Graves' disease)
- Genetic factors
- Thyroid adenomas
- Toxic multinodular goiter
- Increased TSH secretions
- Precipitating factors—excessive dietary intake of iodine and stress can worsen latent hyperthyroidism

What to look for

- Enlarged thyroid (goiter)
- Excitability or nervousness, mood swings

- Heat intolerance and sweating
- Weight loss despite increased appetite
- Frequent bowel movements
- Palpitations
- Hypertension
- Dyspnea on exertion and at rest
- Exophthalmos (classic sign but absent in many patients)
- Difficulty concentrating
- Fine tremor, shaky handwriting, clumsiness
- Weakness, fatigue, and muscle atrophy

How it's treated

- Antithyroid drugs to treat new-onset Graves' disease (spontaneous remission possible) and to correct thyrotoxic state in preparation for radioactive iodine (^{131}I) treatment or surgery
- Thyroid hormone antagonists, including propylthiouracil and methimazole, to block thyroid hormone synthesis
- Beta-adrenergic blocker (propranolol) until antithyroid drugs reach their full effect to manage tachycardia and other peripheral effects of excessive hypersympathetic activity
- Iodine preparations (potassium iodine, ^{131}I) to decrease thyroid gland's capacity for hormone production
- Subtotal thyroidectomy (for those who refuse or aren't candidates for ^{131}I treatment) to decrease thyroid gland's capacity for hormone production
- Lifelong, regular medical supervision to treat hypothyroidism, which develops in most patients after surgery (sometimes several years later)

This is intense

Managing thyroid storm

Thyroid storm, an acute, severe exacerbation of poorly controlled hyperthyroidism, is a medical emergency in which life-threatening cardiac, hepatic, or renal consequences can occur. It may be precipitated by stressors, such as infection, surgery, pregnancy, and diabetic ketoacidosis. If your patient develops thyroid storm, follow these guidelines:

• Monitor blood pressure and cardiac rate and rhythm.
• Administer I.V. beta blockers (such as propranolol) as ordered to block sympathetic effects.
• Monitor temperature and treat high fever.
• Monitor intake and output to ensure adequate hydration following vomiting, diaphoresis, and renal effects.
• Avoid excessive palpation of the thyroid.
• Monitor neurologic status.
• Administer antithyroid drug.
• Administer iodide preparation to block release of thyroid hormone.
• Administer corticosteroid to replace depleted cortical levels and support circulation.
• Administer sedation as necessary for irritability and hyperkinesis.
• Treat precipitating cause or stressor.

Hypothyroidism, adult

- Results from hypothalamic, pituitary, or thyroid insufficiency or resistance to thyroid hormone
- Can progress to life-threatening myxedema coma

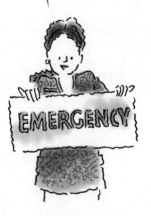

I see, I see

Understanding hypothyroidism

Malfunction of thyroid gland, hypothalamus, or pituitary

Thyroid malfunction	Hypothalamus malfunction	Pituitary malfunction
Lack of negative feedback on pituitary and hypothalamus	Low thyroid hormone, TSH, and TRH levels	No negative feedback to hypothalamus on its release by TSH or thyroid hormone
Low thyroid hormone levels; high TSH and TRH levels		Low thyroid hormone levels

What causes it

- Autoimmune disease (Hashimoto's thyroiditis)
- Overuse of antithyroid drugs
- Thyroidectomy
- Malfunction of pituitary gland
- Radiation therapy (particularly with ^{131}I)

What to look for

- Early signs and symptoms
  - Fatigue
  - Menstrual changes
  - Hypercholesterolemia
  - Forgetfulness

- Sensitivity to cold
- Unexplained weight gain
- Constipation
- Later signs and symptoms
  - Decreasing mental stability
  - Dry, flaky, inelastic skin
  - Puffy face, hands, and feet
  - Hoarseness
  - Periorbital edema, upper eyelid droop
  - Dry, sparse hair and thick brittle nails
  - Cardiovascular changes (decreased cardiac output, bradycardia)
- Myxedema coma following stress in prolonged or severe hypothyroidism

How it's treated

- Gradual thyroid hormone replacement (with synthetic T4 and, occasionally, triiodothyronine)
- High-bulk, low-calorie diet to maintain adequate nutritional status
- Cathartics and stool softeners (as needed) to maintain bowel function
- Surgical excision, chemotherapy, or radiation to reduce the size of or remove a tumor
- Lifelong hormone replacement and routine monitoring

Irritable bowel syndrome (IBS)

- Benign condition that has no anatomic abnormality or inflammatory component

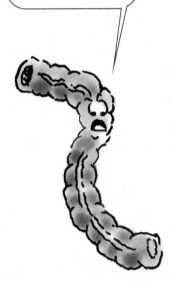

I see, I see

Understanding IBS

In IBS, the entire colon appears to react to stimuli, causing abnormally strong contractions of the intestinal smooth muscle in response to distention, irritants, or stress. Visceral hypersensitivity and altered colonic motility are the mechanisms involved.

Autonomic nervous system fails to produce alternating contractions and relaxations that propel stool smoothly toward the rectum, resulting in constipation, diarrhea, or both.

Constipation	**Diarrhea**	**Mixed symptoms**
Spasmodic intestinal contractions set up partial obstruction by trapping gas and stool.	Eating or cholinergic stimulation triggers contents of small intestine to rush into large intestine (in patients with dramatically increased intestinal motility).	If further spasms trap liquid stool, intestinal mucosa absorbs water from the stool, leaving them dry, hard, and difficult to pass.
Distention, bloating, gas pain, and constipation occur.	Dumping of watery stool and irritation of mucosa occurs, which results in diarrhea.	Pattern of alternating diarrhea and constipation occurs.

What causes it

- Psychological stress (most common)
- Ingestion of irritants (coffee, raw fruit or vegetables)
- Lactose intolerance

- Abuse of laxatives
- Hormonal changes (menstruation)
- Diverticular disease
- Colon cancer

What to look for

- Complaints of cramping, lower abdominal pain relieved by defecation or passage of flatus
- Pain that intensifies 1 to 2 hours after a meal
- Constipation alternating with diarrhea (one is more dominant)
- Mucus passed through rectum from altered secretion in intestines
- Abdominal distention, bloating, and flatulence

How it's treated

- Supportive treatment or avoidance of known irritant to relieve symptoms
- Stress-relief measures, counseling, and mild anti-anxiety agents to decrease colon response to stimuli
- Application of heat to abdomen to relieve spasms and pain
- Antispasmodics to treat cramping
- High-fiber diet to prevent constipation

For diarrhea-dominant IBS

- Bulking agents to reduce episodes of diarrhea and minimize effect of nonpropulsive colonic contractions
- Loperamide to reduce urgency and fecal soiling in patients with persistent diarrhea
- Alosetron (for severe IBS unresponsive to conventional therapy) to relieve pain, decrease urgency, and reduce stool frequency
- Bowel training (if cause is chronic laxative abuse) to regain muscle control

For constipation-dominant IBS

• Cautious use of laxatives to prevent dependency

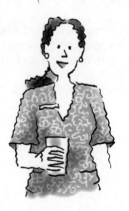

Leukemia, chronic

- Group of malignant disorders characterized by abnormal proliferation of WBC precursors or blasts
- Chronic lymphocytic leukemia (CLL)—uncontrollable spread of small, abnormal lymphocytes in lymphoid tissue, blood, and bone marrow
  - Usually progresses slowly and is common in the elderly
  - Treatment focused on symptom management, not cure
- Chronic myelogenous leukemia (CML)—abnormal overgrowth of granulocytic precursors (myeloblasts, promyelocytes, metamyelocytes, and myelocytes) in bone marrow, blood, and body tissues
  - Most common in young and middle-aged adults
  - Progresses to crisis or acute phase

I see, I see

Understanding leukemia

Leukemias cause an abnormal proliferation of WBCs and suppression of other blood components. Leukemia is characterized by the malignant proliferation of WBC precursors (blasts) in bone marrow or lymph tissue and by their accumulation in peripheral blood, bone marrow, and body tissues. In chronic forms of leukemia, disease onset occurs insidiously, commonly with no symptoms.

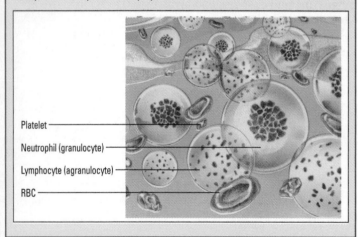

Platelet

Neutrophil (granulocyte)

Lymphocyte (agranulocyte)

RBC

What causes it
• Exact cause unknown

Risk factors
• Viral or genetic factors
• Exposure to ionizing radiation and chemicals

What to look for

- White blood cell count abnormalities
- Anemia
  - Fatigue, weakness, decreased exercise tolerance
  - Pallor, dyspnea, tachycardia, palpitations, headache
- Thrombocytopenia
  - Retinal hemorrhage, ecchymoses, hematuria, melena
  - Bleeding gums, nosebleeds, easy bruising
- Abdominal discomfort and pain due to hepatosplenomegaly
- Low-grade fever
- Anorexia, weight loss
- Renal calculi or gouty arthritis from elevated uric acid due to increased cell death
- Lymph node enlargement, opportunistic or prolonged infection
- Edema from lymph node obstruction in CLL
- Macular to nodular skin eruptions in CLL
- Pulmonary infiltrations in CLL
- Sternal and rib tenderness from leukemic infiltrations in CML

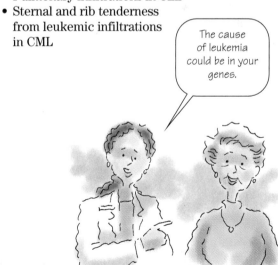

The cause of leukemia could be in your genes.

How it's treated

- Systemic chemotherapy (varies according to type of leukemia) to eradicate leukemic cells and induce remission
- Bone marrow or stem cell transplants (in some cases) to eradicate leukemic cells and induce remission
- Antibiotics, antifungals, antiviral therapy to prevent or control infection
- Immune system support with interferon in CML
- Platelet and RBC transfusions to treat anemia and prevent bleeding; bleeding precautions
- Local radiation to reduce organ size (if leukemia causes obstruction or organ impairment)
- Psychological support to help the patient and family deal with the diagnosis
- Palliative and supportive care for those refractory to chemotherapy or in terminal phase of disease
- Allopurinol to prevent or treat hyperuricemia

Lung cancer

- Development of neoplasm, usually within wall or epithelium of bronchial tree
- Most common types: epidermoid (squamous cell) carcinoma, small cell (oat cell) carcinoma, adenocarcinoma, and large cell (anaplastic) carcinoma

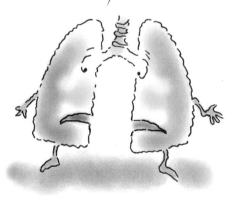

It's hard to believe that lung cancer usually begins with the transformation of a single cell within the wall or epithelium of the bronchial tree.

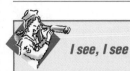

I see, I see

Understanding lung cancer

Lung cancer usually begins with the transformation of one epithelial cell within the patient's airway. Although the exact cause of such change remains unclear, some lung cancers originating in the bronchi may be more vulnerable to injuries from carcinogens.

As the tumor grows, it can partially or completely obstruct the airway, resulting in lobar collapse distal to the tumor. Early metastasis may occur to other thoracic structures as well.

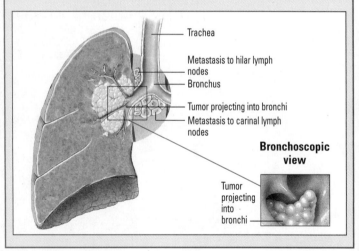

Trachea

Metastasis to hilar lymph nodes

Bronchus

Tumor projecting into bronchi

Metastasis to carinal lymph nodes

Bronchoscopic view

Tumor projecting into bronchi

What causes it

- Inhalation of carcinogenic and industrial air pollutants
- Cigarette smoking
- Genetic predisposition

What to look for

- Usually no symptoms in early stages
- Later symptoms related to cancer cell type and site of metastasis
  - Smoker's cough, hoarseness, wheezing, dyspnea, hemoptysis, and chest or shoulder pain
  - Atelectasis, pneumonitis
  - Unilateral diaphragm paralysis
  - Fever, weakness
  - Anorexia, weight loss
  - Gynecomastia
  - Joint pain
  - Dysphagia
  - Venous distention; facial, neck, and chest edema

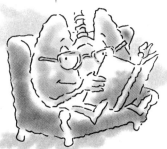

There are several options for treating lung cancer, including surgery, radiation, and chemotherapy.

How it's treated

- Surgical excision of carcinoma; may include partial removal of lung (wedge resection, segmental resection, lobectomy, radical lobectomy) or total removal (pneumonectomy, radical pneumonectomy) to remove tumor
- Preoperative radiation therapy to reduce tumor bulk and allow for surgical resection
- Radiation therapy (recommended for stage I and stage II lesions if surgery is contraindicated; for stage III lesions when disease is confined to involved hemithorax and ipsilateral supraclavicular lymph nodes) to destroy any cancer cells
- Postsurgical radiation therapy (delayed until 1 month after surgery to allow wound to heal, then directed to part of

chest most likely to develop metastasis) to destroy any re-
maining cancer cells
- Chemotherapy to induce regression of tumor or prevent
  metastasis
- Laser therapy (through bronchoscope) to destroy local tu-
  mors
- Smoking cessation
- Nutritional and psychosocial support

Lupus erythematosus

- Inflammatory disorder of the connective tissue
- Discoid type: affects only the skin
- Systemic type (SLE): affects multiple organ systems
- Recurrent remissions and exacerbations

Lupus is a chronic inflammatory disorder of the connective tissue believed to be caused by autoimmunity and triggered by many factors.

I see, I see

Understanding systemic lupus erythematosus

Systemic lupus erythematosus is a chronic inflammatory autoimmune disorder of connective tissue that affects multiple organ systems. It's characterized by recurring remissions and exacerbations.

Immune dysregulation in the form of autoimmunity

▼

B-cell hyperactivity, causing body to produce antibodies against its own cell components

▼

Activation of immune response by formed antigen-antibody complexes

▼

Production of antibodies against many different tissue components (red blood cells, neutrophils, platelets, lymphocytes) or almost any organ or body tissue

▼

Widespread degeneration of connective tissue

▼

Possible cardiovascular, renal, or neurologic complications; severe bacterial infections

What causes it
- Unknown
  - Genetic defect suspected
  - Autoimmunity thought to be prime cause
- Triggered or aggravated by stress, infections, sunlight or ultraviolet light exposure, immunization, pregnancy, and certain drugs

What to look for

- May be insidious and follow no clinical pattern
- Fever, chills
- Weight loss, anorexia
- Malaise and fatigue
- Rash (erythematous in areas of light exposure, classic facial butterfly rash)
- Polyarthralgia
- Vasculitis, Raynaud's phenomenon
- Patchy alopecia and mucous membrane ulcers
- Lymph node enlargement
- Headache, irritability, depression
- Abdominal pain, nausea, vomiting, diarrhea or constipation
- Anemia, leukopenia, thrombocytopenia, and elevated ESR

How it's treated

- Nonsteroidal anti-inflammatory drugs to control arthritis symptoms
- Corticosteroids for skin lesions and systemic symptoms
- Antihypertensive drugs and diet modification with renal disease
- Cytotoxic drugs, dialysis, or kidney transplant for severe kidney involvement

Lyme disease

- Multisystemic disorder caused by *Borrelia burgdorferi* (spirochete transmitted through tick bite)
- Primarily occurs in areas inhabited by small deer ticks (*Ixodes dammini*)
- Typically manifests in three stages
  - Early localized stage
  - Early disseminated stage (weeks to months after bite)
  - Late stage (weeks to years after bite)

Lyme disease is transmitted through tick bites, primarily in grassy or shrubby, wooded areas inhabited by deer.

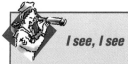

I see, I see

Understanding Lyme disease

A multisystemic disorder caused by the spirochete *B. burgdorferi,* Lyme disease is transmitted to humans by the bite of the minute deer tick *Ixodes dammini* or another tick in the Ixodidae family.

> Tick injects spirochete-laden saliva into host's bloodstream.

> After incubating for 3 to 32 days, spirochetes migrate outward, causing characteristic red macule or papule rash (erythema chronicum migrans).

> Spirochetes disseminate to other skin sites or organs through bloodstream or lymph system.

> Spriochetes may survive for years in joints, or they may trigger inflammatory response in host and die.

What causes it

- Infestation of spirochete *B. burgdorferi* resulting from tick bite (injects spirochete-laden saliva into bloodstream or deposits fecal matter on skin)

What to look for

Early localized stage

- Distinctive red rash that appears as target or bull's eye, commonly at the site of the bite; feels hot and itchy
- Conjunctivitis, diffuse urticaria
- Flulike symptoms: fever, chills, myalgias, headache, stiff neck; malaise, sore throat, dry cough
- Regional lymphadenopathy

Early disseminated stage
- Peripheral and cranial neuropathy; facial palsy
- Carditis, conduction disturbances, ventricular dysfunction

Persistent infection stage
- Chronic neurologic problems
- Migrating musculoskeletal pain
- Frank arthritis with marked joint swelling
- Recurrent attacks preceding chronic arthritis

How it's treated
- Antibiotics to treat infection
  - Early localized disease: doxycycline or amoxicillin for 3 to 4 weeks, or cefuroxime axetil or erythromycin if patient is allergic to penicillin or tetracycline
  - Late disease: I.V. ceftriaxone or penicillin for 4 or more weeks
- Anti-inflammatory agents to treat arthritis
- Close monitoring for ptosis, strabismus, and diplopia to detect signs of increased intracranial pressure and cranial nerve involvement
- Monitoring of heart rate and rhythm to detect arrhythmias

Macular degeneration

- Atrophy or degeneration of the macular region of the retina
- Two age-related types
  - Dry or atrophic: slow, progressive, mild vision loss; can develop into wet form
  - Wet, exudative: progressive visual distortion leading to vision loss

What causes it

- Hardening and obstruction of retinal arteries
- Formation of new abnormal blood vessels that grow and leak, obscuring central vision in wet form

Risk factors

- Family history
- Cigarette smoking

What to look for

- Visual changes
  - Straight lines that become distorted
  - Blurring or blank area that appears in the center of a printed page (central scotoma)
  - Difficulty recognizing faces
  - More light required for reading and other tasks

How it's treated

- Laser photocoagulation to destroy new, abnormal blood vessels
- Photodynamic laser therapy of wet form to close abnormal blood vessels
- Nutrition support—vitamins B and C, beta-carotene, and zinc to slow progression of dry degeneration
- Antivascular endothelial growth factor (VEGF) drug therapy to block growth of abnormal vessels
- Vision aids

Vision problems should be addressed sooner rather than later to avoid loss of sight.

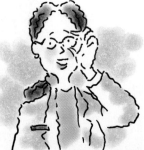

Malignant melanoma

- Neoplasm arising from melanocytes and characterized by enlargement of skin lesion or nevus accompanied by changes in color, inflammation, soreness, itching, ulceration, bleeding, or textural changes
- Common sites: head and neck (men), legs (women), and back (those exposed to excessive sunlight); up to 70% arise from preexisting nevus
- Classified as superficial spreading melanoma, nodular malignant melanoma, lentigo maligna melanoma, and acral-lentiginous melanoma
- About 10 times more common among white populations

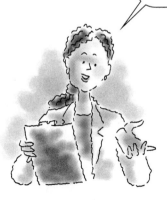

A malignant melanoma is usually marked by changes in size, color, and texture and can be accompanied by inflammation, soreness, itching, ulceration, and bleeding.

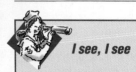

I see, I see

How malignant melanoma develops

A malignant neoplasm that arises from melanocytes, malignant melanoma can arise on normal skin or from an existing mole. If not treated promptly, it can spread through the lymphatic and vascular system and metastasize to the regional lymph nodes, skin, liver, lungs, and central nervous system. These illustrations show a cross-section of a malignant melanoma and its defining characteristics.

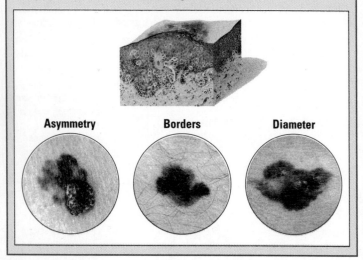

Asymmetry   **Borders**   **Diameter**

What causes it

- Excessive exposure to ultraviolet (UV) light
- History of blistering sunburn before age 20
- Skin type
  - Whites: typically those with blond or red hair, fair skin, and blue eyes who are prone to sunburn and of Celtic or Scandinavian descent

- Blacks: usually arises in lightly pigmented areas (palms, plantar surface of feet, fingernails and toenails, or mucous membranes)
- Genetic or autoimmune factors
- Hormonal factors (pregnancy may increase risk and exacerbate growth)

Risk factors
- Family history
- History of melanoma (recurrence 10 times more likely)
- Occupational history

What to look for

- Skin lesion or nevus enlargement, color change, inflammation or soreness, itching, ulceration, bleeding, textural change, or pigment regression of surrounding tissue

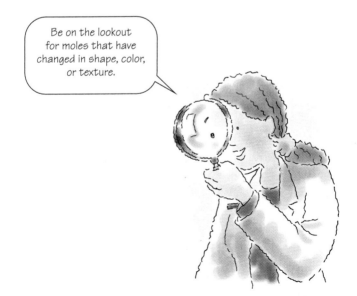

Be on the lookout for moles that have changed in shape, color, or texture.

How it's treated

- Surgical resection to remove tumor (extent depends on size and location of primary tumor; could require skin graft)
- Regional lymphadenectomy to help prevent metastasis
- Chemotherapy or biotherapy (for deep primary lesions) to eliminate or reduce number of tumor cells
- Radiation therapy or gene therapy for metastatic disease
- Long-term follow-up to detect metastasis and recurrences
- Patient teaching and recommendation of sun block use and other protection to help prevent recurrence

Head of the class

Minimizing sun exposure

To help your patient minimize exposure to the sun's harmful effects, provide these guidelines:
• Know that protection should begin in childhood for best effect.
• Use a sunscreen that contains para-aminobenzoic acid and has a sun protection factor (SPF) of 15 or higher.
• Apply sunscreen 30 minutes before going outside.
• Reapply every 2 to 3 hours, or more frequently with heavy perspiration, exercise, or swimming.
• Keep sunscreen available in the car and at work, not just at home.
• Wear protective clothing, such as a wide-brimmed hat, long sleeves, and sunglasses with total UV protection.
• Don't rely on tree shade or overcast sky to provide protection from ultraviolet rays.
• Remember that sun reflects off of water, snow, and sand, intensifying its effects.
• Avoid outdoor activities during the strongest sun hours of 10 a.m. to 3 p.m.
• Check with your healthcare provider or pharmacist about possible phototropic (sensitizing) effects of prescription and over-the-counter medications.
• Avoid sunlamps and tanning parlors or booths.

Mitral insufficiency

- Inadequate closing of mitral valve
- Backflow of blood from left ventricle to right atrium during systole

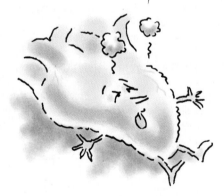

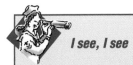

I see, I see

Understanding mitral insufficiency

An abnormality of the mitral leaflets, mitral annulus, chordae tendineae, papillary muscles, left atrium, or left ventricle can lead to mitral insufficiency. Blood from the left ventricle flows back into the left atrium during systole; the atrium enlarges to accommodate the backflow. As a result, the left ventricle also dilates to accommodate the increased blood volume from the atrium and to compensate for diminishing cardiac output. Ventricular hypertrophy and increased end-diastolic pressure result in increased pulmonary artery pressure, eventually leading to left-sided and right-sided heart failure.

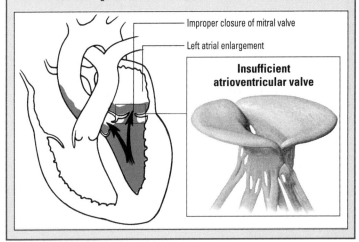

Improper closure of mitral valve

Left atrial enlargement

Insufficient atrioventricular valve

What causes it

- Rheumatic fever
- Mitral valve prolapse
- Hypertrophic obstructive cardiomyopathy
- Myocardial infarction

- Ruptured chordae tendineae
- Transposition of great arteries

What to look for

- Holosystolic murmur at apex of heart
- Angina from impaired coronary circulation
- Orthopnea, dyspnea, crackles, heart failure
- Fatigue
- Peripheral edema, hepatomegaly and jugular vein distention
- Tachycardia and palpitations

How it's treated

- Digoxin, low-sodium diet, diuretics, vasodilators, and especially ACE inhibitors to treat left-sided heart failure
- Oxygen (in acute situations) to increase oxygenation
- Anticoagulants to prevent thrombus formation around diseased or replaced valves
- Prophylactic antibiotics before and after surgery or dental care to prevent endocarditis
- Nitroglycerin to relieve angina
- Antiarrhythmics to control heart rate and rhythm
- Valve replacement or repair to control symptoms

Mitral stenosis

- Narrowing of mitral valve orifice
- Valve leaflets thickened by fibrosis and calcification

I see, I see

Understanding mitral stenosis

In mitral stenosis, narrowing of the mitral valve by valvular abnormalities, fibrosis, or calcification obstructs blood flow from the left atrium to the left ventricle. Left atrial volume and pressure rise and the chamber dilates. Greater resistance to blood flow causes pulmonary hypertension, right ventricular hypertrophy, and right-sided heart failure. Inadequate filling of the left ventricle results in low cardiac output.

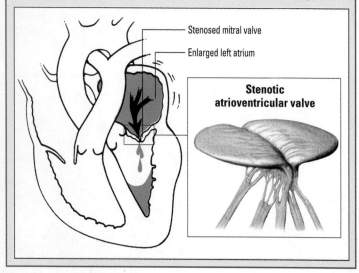

Stenosed mitral valve

Enlarged left atrium

Stenotic atrioventricular valve

What causes it

- Rheumatic fever
- Congenital abnormalities
- Atrial myxoma
- Endocarditis

- Adverse effect of fenfluramine and phentermine diet drug combination (This drug combination has been removed from the U.S. drug market.)

What to look for

- Opening snap and diastolic murmur
- Angina
- Dyspnea on exertion, paroxysmal nocturnal dyspnea, orthopnea, and heart failure
- Weakness and fatigue
- Tachycardia, arrhythmias, and palpitations
- Peripheral edema, jugular vein distention, hepatomegaly

How it's treated

- Digoxin, low-sodium diet, diuretics, vasodilators, and especially ACE inhibitors to treat left-sided heart failure
- Oxygen (in acute situations) to increase oxygenation
- Anticoagulants to prevent thrombus formation around diseased or replaced valves
- Prophylactic antibiotics before and after surgery or dental care to prevent endocarditis
- Nitrates to relieve angina
- Beta-adrenergic blockers or digoxin to slow the ventricular rate in atrial fibrillation or atrial flutter

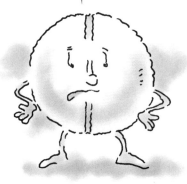

Prophylactic drugs should be used before and after surgery or dental care to prevent endocarditis.

- Cardioversion to convert atrial fibrillation to sinus rhythm
- Balloon valvuloplasty to enlarge the orifice of a stenotic mitral valve
- Prosthetic valve to replace a damaged valve that can't be repaired

Multiple sclerosis

- Characterized by progressive demyelination of white matter of brain and spinal cord with periods of exacerbation and remission
- Transient symptoms lasting for hours or weeks and varying from day to day without pattern
- Major cause of chronic disability in young adults ages 20 to 40

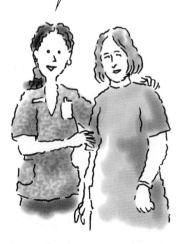

I see, I see

How myelin breaks down

Myelin speeds electrical impulses to the brain for interpretation. This lipoprotein complex protects the neuron's axon much like the insulation on an electrical wire. Its high electrical resistance and low capacitance allow the myelin to conduct nerve impulses from one node of Ranvier to the next.

Myelin is susceptible to injury. The sheath becomes inflamed, and the membrane layers break down into smaller components that become well-circumscribed plaques. This process is called *demyelination*.

The damaged myelin sheath can't conduct normally. The partial loss or dispersion of the action potential causes neurologic dysfunction.

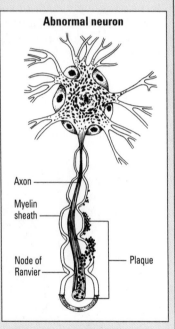

Abnormal neuron

Axon

Myelin sheath

Node of Ranvier

Plaque

What causes it

- Exact cause unknown
- Possibly slow-acting or latent viral infection that triggers autoimmune response or environmental or genetic factors
- Conditions that may precede onset or exacerbation: emotional stress, fatigue (physical or emotional), pregnancy, and acute respiratory infections

What to look for

- Initially, vision problems (such as diplopia, blurred vision, optic neuritis, ocular muscle paralysis, and nystagmus) and sensory impairment (such as numbness and tingling, loss of balance)
- Weakness and paralysis of one or more limbs, spasticity, hyperreflexia, intention tremor, and gait ataxia
- Urinary incontinence, frequency, urgency, and frequent infections; bowel disturbances
- Mood swings, irritability, euphoria and depression
- Dizziness
- Heat sensitivity
- Impaired concentration or memory
- Speech dysfunction and dysphagia

How it's treated

- I.V. methylprednisolone followed by oral therapy to reduce edema of myelin sheath (speeds recovery from acute attacks)
- Immunotherapy (interferon, glatiramer, mitoxantrone) to reduce frequency and severity of relapses and possibly slow central nervous system (CNS) damage
- Pain management related to neuralgia and spasticity
- Amantadine, modafinil, and antidepressants to help manage fatigue
- Low-dose tricyclic antidepressants, phenytoin, or carbamazepine to manage sensory symptoms (pain, numbness, burning, and tingling)
- Beta-adrenergic blockers, sedatives, or diuretics to alleviate tremor
- Increased fiber intake, use of bulking agents, or bowel-training strategies (daily suppositories and rectal stimulation) to help manage bowel problems
- Baclofen or tizanidine orally to treat mild to moderate spasticity; botulinum toxin injections, intrathecal baclofen (in-

jections or pump implantations), nerve blocks, or surgery to treat severe spasticity
- Stretching and range-of-motion (ROM) exercises (coupled with correct positioning) to relieve spasticity resulting from opposing muscle groups relaxing and contracting at the same time
- Frequent rest, aerobic exercise, and cooling (air conditioning, breezes, water sprays) to help minimize fatigue
- Anticholinergic drugs to treat bladder dysfunction, bladder training, catheterization (self, indwelling, suprapubic)
- Adaptive devices, occupational and physical therapy to assist with motor dysfunction
- Speech therapy to treat dysarthria

Muscular dystrophy

- Group of congenital disorders characterized by progressive symmetrical wasting of skeletal muscles without neural or sensory defects
- Degenerated muscle fibers replaced by fat and connective tissue
- Initially affects the leg and pelvic muscles but eventually spreads to the involuntary muscles

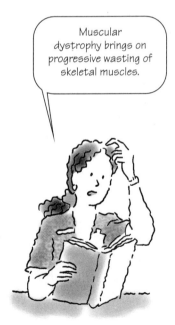

What causes it

- Genetic disorder

What to look for

- Insidious onset
- Signs and symptoms that vary by specific muscular dystrophy disorder
- Overdeveloped calf muscles
- Abnormal gait, lordosis, and poor balance
- Contractures, scoliosis
- Intermittent oscillation of the irises in response to light
- Tachycardia and ECG changes due to cardiac muscle weakening
- Abnormal or absent facial movements

How it's treated

- No treatment to stop its progression
- Supportive treatment with occupational and physical therapy and assistive devices
- Surgery to correct contractures
- Prednisone to improve muscle strength and slow degeneration
- Nutritional support to prevent obesity and constipation
- Pulmonary care to prevent complications due to immobility and respiratory muscle involvement
- Genetic counseling for family members
- Referral to Muscular Dystrophy Association

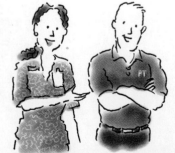

People with muscular dystrophy benefit from physical and occupational therapy.

Myasthenia gravis

- Disease that causes sporadic but progressive weakness and abnormal fatigability of striated (skeletal) muscles
- Typically affects muscles innervated by cranial nerves (face, lips, tongue, neck, throat) but may affect any muscle group
- Unpredictable course of exacerbations and remissions

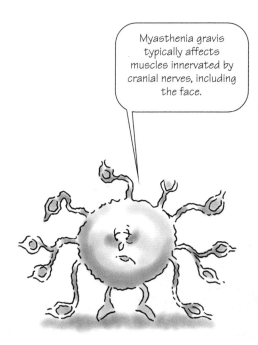

Myasthenia gravis typically affects muscles innervated by cranial nerves, including the face.

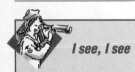

I see, I see

Understanding myasthenia gravis

During normal neuromuscular transmission, a motor nerve impulse travels to a motor nerve terminal, stimulating release of a chemical neurotransmitter called *acetylcholine*. When acetylcholine diffuses across the synapse, receptor sites in the motor end-plate react and depolarize the muscle fiber. Depolarization spreads through the muscle fiber, causing muscle contraction.

In myasthenia gravis, antibodies attach to the acetylcholine receptor sites. They block, destroy, and weaken these sites, leaving them insensitive to acetylcholine, thereby blocking neuromuscular transmission.

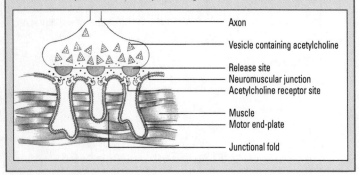

- Axon
- Vesicle containing acetylcholine
- Release site
- Neuromuscular junction
- Acetylcholine receptor site
- Muscle
- Motor end-plate
- Junctional fold

What causes it

- Exact cause unknown
- May result from autoimmune response, ineffective acetylcholine release, or inadequate muscle fiber response to acetylcholine

What to look for

- First signs: weak eye closure, ptosis, and diplopia

- Progressive skeletal muscle weakness and fatigability; may eventually cause paralysis
- Muscles strongest in the morning but weaken throughout the day, especially after exercise; rest periods help
- Blank, expressionless face
- Nasal vocal tones; difficulty chewing and swallowing
- Frequent nasal regurgitation of fluids
- Difficulty breathing and predisposition to respiratory tract infections if respiratory muscles are involved

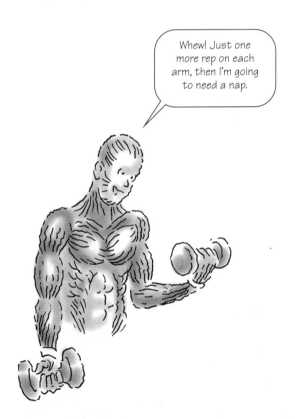

This is intense

Myasthenic crisis and cholinergic crisis

Myasthenic crisis is an acute exacerbation of the muscular weakness that occurs in myasthenia gravis. It can be triggered by infection, surgery, emotional stress, drug interaction, alcohol ingestion, temperature extremes, or pregnancy. Insufficient anticholinesterase medication can also cause myasthenic crisis. Signs and symptoms of myasthenic crisis include:

- anxiety, restlessness, irritability
- respiratory distress progressing to apnea
- dysarthria, dysphagia
- extreme fatigue
- fever
- inability to move jaw or raise one or both eyelids
- increased muscular weakness.

Cholinergic crisis results from an overdose of, or toxicity to, anticholinesterase agents used to treat myasthenia. Typical signs and symptoms of cholinergic crisis include:

- increasing anxiety and apprehension
- anorexia, nausea, vomiting, abdominal cramps
- excessive salivation
- sweating
- fasciculation (twitching) around the eyes
- muscle cramps and spasms
- increasing muscle weakness
- dysarthria, increasing dysphagia
- respiratory distress.

Both myasthenic and cholinergic crises are emergency situations that require immediate intervention. When caring for a patient who experiences one of these crises, follow these guidelines:

- Notify the physician immediately.
- Maintain a patent airway; provide respiratory support as needed, including oxygen therapy or assisted ventilation.

Myasthenic crisis and cholinergic crisis *(continued)*

• Assist with the administration of edrophonium I.V.
• Provide supportive care, including parenteral fluids, antibiotics (if the crisis was due to infection), enteral feedings, or the insertion of an indwelling urinary catheter.
• Provide emotional support and be sure to explain all the events as they're happening to help allay some of the patient's fears and anxieties.

How it's treated

- Anticholinesterase drugs to counteract fatigue, muscle weakness
- Immunosuppressant therapy (corticosteroids, azathioprine, cyclosporine, and cyclophosphamide) used progressively to decrease immune response toward acetylcholine receptors at neuromuscular junction
- Immunoglobulin G (during acute relapses) or plasmapheresis (in severe exacerbations) to suppress immune system
- Thymectomy to remove thymomas and induce remission in adult-onset myasthenia

- Immediate hospitalization, respiratory support, and discontinuation of anticholinesterase drugs to treat myasthenic crisis until respiratory function improves
- Tracheotomy, mechanical ventilation, and suctioning to improve respiratory function and remove secretions for treatment of acute exacerbations
- Referral to Myasthenia Gravis Foundation for support and information about the disease, lifestyle changes, and nutrition

N-Z

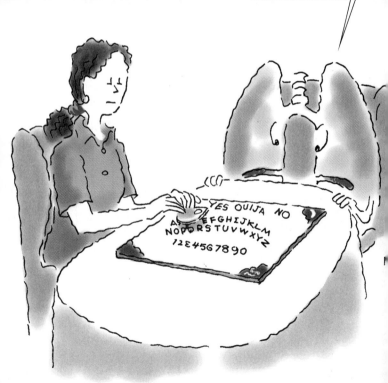

Neurogenic bladder

- Any bladder dysfunction caused by an interruption of normal bladder innervation
- Can be spastic (hypertonic, reflex, or automatic) or flaccid (hypotonic, atonic, nonreflex, or autonomous)

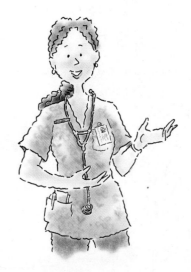

A neurogenic bladder can be spastic or flaccid.

What causes it

- Spinal cord disease or trauma
- Cerebral disorders such as stroke, brain tumor, Parkinson's disease, multiple sclerosis, or dementia
- Neuropathy secondary to diabetes, vascular disease, acute infection, chronic alcoholism, and other disorders
- Metabolic disturbances

What to look for

- Incontinence
- Changes in initiation, interruption of voiding, and inability to empty the bladder completely
- Bladder distention and secondary symptoms of headache, hypertension, and bradycardia
- Loss of sensation of bladder fullness
- Urinary tract infection
- Stone formation
- Renal failure
- Diminished or increased anal sphincter tone, fecal impaction

How it's treated

- Valsalva's maneuver to promote evacuation of bladder
- Credé's method—application of manual pressure over the lower abdomen to promote evacuation of bladder
- Intermittent self-catheterization
- Bethanechol and phenoxybenzamine to facility bladder emptying
- Flavoxate, hyoscyamine, and imipramine to relax and prevent bladder spasms
- Alpha-blocker (tamsulosin, terazosin, doxazosin) to relax urethral sphincter
- Surgery to correct structural impairment
- Implantation of artificial urinary sphincter
- Electrical bladder stimulation when other treatments have not worked

Obesity

- Excess of body fat
- Generally 20% above ideal body weight
- Body mass index of 30 or more

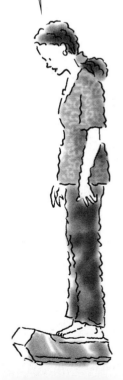

What causes it

- Excessive calorie intake
- Inadequate expenditure of energy

Risk factors

- Gender (more common in women)
- Age
- Pregnancy
- Hypothalamic dysfunction
- Genetic predisposition
- Abnormal nutrient absorption
- Hormonal imbalances
  - GI hormones
  - Growth hormones
  - Insulin
- Lower socioeconomic status
- Environmental factors such as learned activity and eating habits
- Psychological factors such as depression, stress, and emotional upset, which can promote excessive eating

What to look for

- Indication of obesity by standard height and weight table
- Body mass index of 30 or more
- Elevated total body fat by subcutaneous fat fold measurements
- Associated signs and symptoms
  - Snoring and sleep apnea
  - Gastroesophageal reflux disease
  - Arthritic and joint pain
  - Poor body image, poor self-esteem, and depression
- Co-morbidities
  - Hypertension, stroke, and cardiovascular disease
  - Diabetes
  - Gallbladder disease
  - Renal disease

– Osteoarthritis
– Respiratory difficulties
– Colon and endometrial cancer

How it's treated

- Dietary and nutritional counseling
- Supervised exercise program
- Behavior modification; hypnosis in some cases
- Psychotherapy and anti-depressants if appropriate
- Appetite suppressants and lipase inhibitors with careful supervision in addition to overall weight loss program
- Bariatric surgery in selected patients with BMI greater than 35 and at an absolute risk for increased morbidity or premature mortality without weight loss

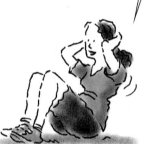

23...24...25...With diet and exercise, obesity can be overcome!

Calculating BMI

Use these steps to calculate body mass index (BMI):
- Multiply weight in pounds by 705.
- Divide this number by height in inches.
- Then divide it by height in inches again.
- Compare results to these standards:
  – 18.5 to 24.9: normal
  – 25 to 29.9: overweight
  – 30 to 39.9: obese
  – 40 or greater: morbidly obese.

Obsessive-compulsive disorder

- Obsession—unwanted recurrent idea, thought, impulse, or image that's intrusive and inappropriate and causes marked anxiety or distress
- Compulsion—ritualistic, repetitive, and involuntary defensive behavior or mental act that reduces anxiety, prompting the patient to repeat the behavior
- Compulsions commonly associated with obsessions
- Episodes of remissions and flare-ups usually related to stress
- May be simple or complex and ritualized
- May be overt behaviors (such as hand washing) or mental activities (such as praying or counting)

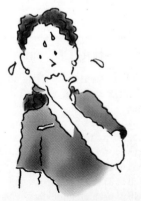

Obsessive-compulsive disorder is a type of anxiety disorder that commonly manifests during periods of overwhelming stress.

What causes it

- Unknown, but other psychological disorders may contribute to its onset
- Possible genetic component
- Possible biologic relationship to strep infections

What to look for

- Repetitive thoughts that cause stress
- Perceived need to achieve perfection
- Repetitive behaviors, which the patient will often attempt to hide to prevent shame or embarrassment
- Impaired social and occupational functioning
- Physical complications of behavior such as dermatitis from compulsive hand washing

How it's treated

- Benzodiazepine or antidepressants
- Behavior modification therapies
- Relaxation techniques
- Support groups to decrease patient isolation

Memory jogger

To help the patient cope with OCD, remember the word COPING.

C: Concerns and feelings are discussed.

O: Offer a structured routine that allows time for rituals.

P: Practice thought-stopping skills.

I: Initiate a behavioral contract to decrease rituals and reward non-ritualistic behaviors.

N: Nurture effective ways to problem-solve stressful situations.

G: Get the patient to perform relaxation techniques.

Obstructive sleep apnea syndrome

- Disruption in breathing during sleep that lasts at least 10 seconds and typically occurs more than 5 times in 1 hour
- Incidence: increases with age

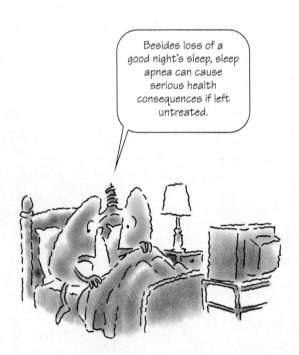

I see, I see

What happens in obstructive sleep apnea

Skeletal muscles relax during sleep.

Tongue and other anatomic structures of head and neck become displaced, resulting in obstruction of upper airway even though chest wall continues to move.

Absence of breathing increases arterial carbon dioxide levels and lowers pH level.

Stimulation of nervous system occurs and person responds after 10 or more seconds of apnea, correcting the obstruction, and breathing resumes.

Cycle repeats as often as every 5 minutes, affecting patient's ability to get a restful night of sleep.

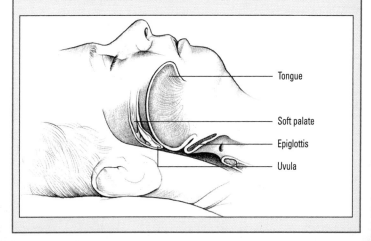

Tongue

Soft palate

Epiglottis

Uvula

What causes it
- Soft palate or tongue obstructing the upper airway

Risk factors
- Obesity
- Large uvula
- Shorter than normal neck
- Enlarged tonsils or adenoids

What to look for
- Snoring
- Observed apnea
- Morning headaches
- Excessive daytime sleepiness
- Intellectual impairment and memory loss
- Cardiorespiratory symptoms, such as hypertension
- Depression, anxiety, mood changes
- Impotence
- Weight gain

How it's treated
- Weight loss
- Smoking cessation
- Change in sleeping position
- Surgical intervention (adenoidectomy, uvulectomy, or reconstruction of the oropharynx)
- Bilevel positive airway pressure system (BiPAP)
- Nasal continuous positive airway pressure system (CPAP)
- Tracheostomy as last resort

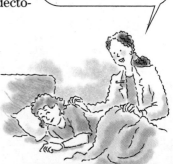

Sometimes just changing the sleeping position can improve obstructive sleep apnea.

Osteoarthritis

- Chronic condition causing deterioration of joint cartilage and formation of reactive new bone
- Usually affects weight-bearing joints

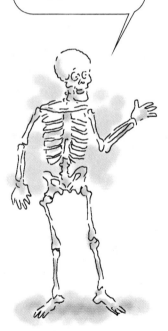

I see, I see

Understanding osteoarthritis

Osteoarthritis occurs as synovial joint cartilage deteriorates, and reactive, new bone forms at the margins and subchondral areas of the joints. Such degeneration results from damage to chondrocytes (cells responsible for binding cartilage). Cartilage normally softens with age, narrowing the joint space. Mechanical injuries can erode articular cartilage, leaving the underlying bone unprotected and causing sclerosis.

Cartilage flakes irritate the synovial lining, which becomes fibrotic and limits joint movement. New bone (osteophyte, or *bone spur*) forms at joint margins as the articular cartilage erodes, causing gross alteration of the bony contours and joint enlargement. This illustration shows how repeated inflammation causes bony enlargement of the distal and proximal interphalangeal joints, called *Heberden's* and *Bouchard's nodes.*

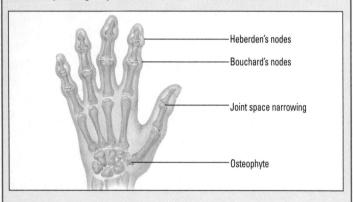

What causes it

Primary osteoarthritis
- Metabolic factors (endocrine disorders such as hyper-parathyroidism) and genetic factors
- Chemical factors (drugs, such as steroids, that stimulate collagen-digesting enzymes in synovial membrane)
- Mechanical factors (repeated stress on joint)

Secondary osteoarthritis
- Trauma (most common cause)
- Congenital deformity
- Obesity

What to look for
- Deep, aching joint pain, particularly after exercise or weight bearing (usually relieved by rest)
- Stiffness in the morning and after exercise (usually relieved by rest)
- Aching associated with weather changes, "grating" of joint during motion, altered gait contractures
- Nodes that eventually become red, swollen, and tender, causing numbness and loss of dexterity

How it's treated
- Exercise to keep joints flexible and improve muscle strength
- Medications (non-NSAIDs, corticosteroids, NSAIDs) to control pain and decrease inflammation as appropriate with patient's medical history
- Glucocorticoid injections for inflamed joints unresponsive to NSAIDs
- Intra-articular injections of hyaluronate to lubricate the joint
- Heat or cold therapy for temporary pain relief
- Joint protection to prevent strain or stress on painful joints and improve activity tolerance

- Surgery (arthroplasty, arthrodesis, osteoplasty, osteotomy) to relieve chronic pain in damaged joints, reconstruct joints, and increase function
- Weight control to prevent extra stress on weight-bearing joints
- Physical therapy and use of assistive devices to improve activities of daily living

Osteoporosis

- Metabolic bone disorder in which rate of bone resorption accelerates while rate of bone formation slows, causing loss of bone mass
- Affected bones abnormally vulnerable to fractures
- May be classified as primary (commonly called post-menopausal osteoporosis) or secondary to other causes

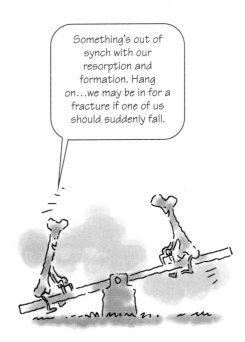

I see, I see

How osteoporosis develops

In osteoporosis, bones weaken as local cells reabsorb bone tissue. Trabecular bone at the core becomes less dense, and cortical bone on the perimeter becomes thinner. Bones affected by this disease lose calcium and phosphate salts and become porous, brittle, and abnormally vulnerable to fractures.

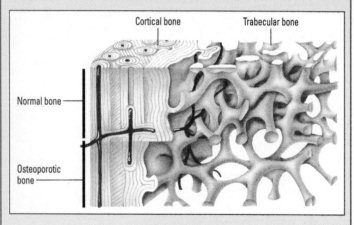

Cortical bone Trabecular bone

Normal bone

Osteoporotic bone

What causes it

- Unknown (primary disease), but linked to many risk factors
- Prolonged therapy involving steroids or heparin
- Total immobility or disuse of bone
- Osteogenesis imperfecta (inherited disorder of the connective tissue)
- Medications (aluminum-containing antacids, corticosteroids, anticonvulsants, antidepressants)

Risk factors
- History of fracture (occurring after age 50)
- Decreased bone mass
- Female gender (especially postmenopausal)
- Thinness or small body frame
- Advanced age
- Family history of osteoporosis
- Estrogen deficiency (menopause related)
- Amenorrhea
- Anorexia nervosa
- Low lifetime calcium intake
- Low testosterone level (males)
- Sedentary lifestyle
- Cigarette smoking
- Excessive alcohol use
- Excessive caffeine intake
- History of depression

How it's treated
- Physical therapy (emphasizing gentle exercise and activity) and regular, moderate weight-bearing exercise to slow bone loss and possibly reverse demineralization
- Supportive devices (back brace) to maintain function
- Hormone replacement therapy (estrogen and progesterone) at the lowest effective dose to slow bone loss and prevent fractures (remains controversial; research is ongoing)
- Analgesics and local heat to relieve pain

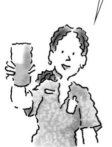

Drink up! The calcium in milk can help prevent osteoporosis.

- Calcium and vitamin D supplements (or a diet rich in calcium and vitamin D) to promote normal bone metabolism
- Bone resorption inhibitor (calcitonin) to reduce bone resorption and slow loss of bone mass
- Bisphosphonates (etidronate, alendronate) to increase bone density and restore lost bone
- Selective estrogen-receptor modulator (raloxifene) to increase bone mineral density
- Parathyroid hormone (teriparatide) to stimulate new bone formation
- Routine monitoring for disease progression

Otitis media, chronic

- Inflammation of the middle ear with effusion or fluid buildup without symptoms of infection
- Often follows an ear infection
- Considered chronic if the fluid remains for more than 3 months
- Majority of cases in children

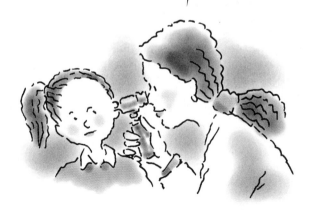

Chronic otitis media commonly follows an ear infection and often causes a popping, ringing, or feeling of fullness or pressure in the ear and, sometimes, temporary hearing loss.

What causes it
- Blockage of Eustachian tubes from lymphoid tissue swelling secondary to a cold, allergy, or infection

What to look for
- Complaints of popping, ringing, or a feeling of fullness or pressure in the ear
- Loss of hearing (usually temporary)
- Delayed speech development
- May be asymptomatic
- History of acute infection

How it's treated
- Without hearing loss—possible delay in treatment to allow further time for fluid reabsorption
- Less than 2 years old or with other chronic disorders—immediate treatment to avoid hearing loss, delayed speech development, and other complications
- Antibiotics to treat acute infection or after prolonged effusion without improvement
- Analgesics for ear pain
- Myringotomy to drain exudate and release pressure
- Tympanoplasty ventilating tubes to equalize pressure on both sides of the tympanic membrane
- Removal of the adenoids and possibly the tonsils to eliminate Eustachian tube blockage

Ovarian cancer

- Highest mortality of all gynecologic cancers
- Most common site of metastatic cancer in women with previously treated breast cancer
- Usually in advanced stage at time of diagnosis due to few presenting signs and symptoms
- Three types
  - Germ cell from the cells that produce oocytes (eggs)
  - Stromal from the connective tissue cells that support the ovary and produce hormones
  - Epithelial from the cells that cover the ovary

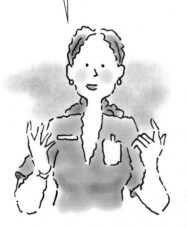

Unfortunately, ovarian cancer usually isn't diagnosed until it's in an advanced stage due to few presenting signs and symptoms. And it has the highest mortality rate of all gynecologic cancers.

What causes it
- Unknown

Risk factors
- Fifth decade of life
- Infertility
- Nulliparity
- Familial history
- Ovarian dysfunction
- Irregular menses
- Possible exposure to asbestos, talc, and industrial pollutants

What to look for
- Early stages—may be asymptomatic or cause vague abdominal discomfort, dyspepsia, and other mild GI disturbances
- Urinary frequency
- Constipation
- Pelvic discomfort
- Abdominal distention, ascites in advanced cases
- Weight loss
- Pain from tumor rupture, torsion, or infection (may mimic appendicitis)
- Feminizing or virilizing effects, depending on tumor type
- Postmenopausal bleeding

Symptoms, when they occur, are often vague or mimic those of other conditions.

How it's treated
- Surgical resection (hysterectomy, unilateral or bilateral salpingo-oophorectomy, depending on the cancer stage)
- Hormone replacement, depending on the patient's age
- Chemotherapy
- Infrequently, radiation therapy

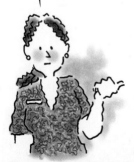

Paget's disease

- Slowly progressive metabolic bone disease
- Osteoclastic phase—initial excessive bone resorption
- Osteoblastic phase—reactive, excessive abnormal bone formation
- Causes deformities of both external contour and internal structure of skeleton
- Causes abnormal bone to impinge on spinal cord or sensory nerve roots, causing pain

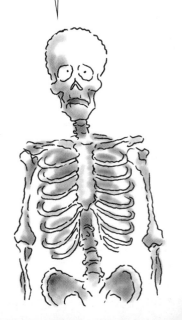

Paget's disease occurs in stages and typically causes skeletal deformities and severe, persistent pain and pathologic fractures...yikes!

What causes it

- Unknown
- Possible viral or genetic factors

What to look for

- Early stages possibly asymptomatic
- Severe and persistent pain
- Impaired movement and muscle weakness
- Kyphosis, barrel chest
- Asymmetrical bowing of the tibia and femur, causing decreased height
- Pathologic fractures with minor trauma
- Blindness and hearing loss with impingement on the cranial nerves
- Headaches
- Congestive heart failure in some cases

How it's treated

- Calcitonin to retard bone resorption
- Bisphosphonates to reduce bone turnover and relieve pain
- Plicamycin, a cytotoxic antibiotic, for severe, resistant cases to decrease calcium, urinary hydroxyproline, and serum alkaline phosphatase levels
- Orthopedic surgery to correct deformities in severe cases, reduce or prevent pathologic fractures, or relieve neurologic impairment
- Analgesics or nonsteroidal anti-inflammatory drugs for pain control
- Physical and occupational therapy and assistive devices to maximize independence

Pancreatitis

- Acute inflammation and fibrosis of the pancreas that causes progressive insufficiency and eventually destroys the pancreas
- Good prognosis when associated with biliary tract disease; poor when associated with alcoholism
- Mortality as high as 60% (with necrosis and hemorrhage)

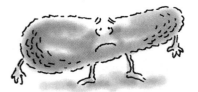

I have a good prognosis when my condition is associated with biliary tract disease...not so good when alcoholism is the source of my worries.

I see, I see

Understanding acute pancreatitis

Acute pancreatitis, which is life-threatening, may be classified as edematous (interstitial) or necrotizing. In both types, inappropriate activation of enzymes causes tissue damage. The mechanism that triggers this activation is unknown; however, conditions associated with it include biliary tract obstruction by gallstones and alcohol abuse.

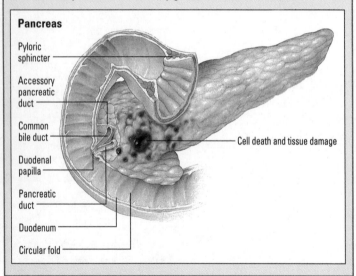

Pancreas

- Pyloric sphincter
- Accessory pancreatic duct
- Common bile duct
- Duodenal papilla
- Pancreatic duct
- Duodenum
- Circular fold
- Cell death and tissue damage

What causes it

- Alcohol abuse
- Hyperparathyroidism
- Hyperlipidemia
- Malnutrition or prolonged fasting
- Heredity (rare)
- Gallstones or biliary tract disease

- Pancreatic cancer
- Trauma
- Peptic ulcers
- Use of certain drugs (glucocorticoids, sulfonamides, chlorothiazide, azthioprine)

What to look for

- Constant dull pain in the midepigastrium, left chest, and back, with acute episodes aggravated by meals and relieved by bending forward
- Anorexia, nausea, vomiting, weight loss
- Hyperglycemia, diabetes
- Bulky, foul-smelling stools
- Anemia
- Tachycardia, hypotension
- Low-grade fever
- Abdominal tenderness and swelling
- Bluish tinge around the navel, bruising of the flanks
- Jaundice

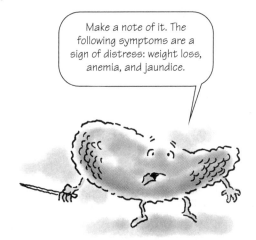

How it's treated

- Alcohol cessation
- Pancreatic enzyme supplements at meals
- Analgesics for pain control
- Low-fat, high-carbohydrate diet
- Antiemetics to alleviate nausea and vomiting
- Histamine antagonists to decrease hydrochloric acid production
- Antibiotics to fight bacterial infections
- Anticholinergics to reduce vagal stimulation, decrease GI motility, and inhibit pancreatic enzyme secretion
- Insulin or oral hypoglycemics to correct hyperglycemia
- Surgery to drain, repair, or remove affected tissue

Panic disorder

- Most severe form of anxiety
- Often begins as response to sudden loss or severe separation anxiety
- May become associated with a specific situation or task
- Can lead to behavior changes and lifestyle restriction from worry over recurrence and its consequences; often exists concurrently with agoraphobia
- Varying frequency and severity; may occur in clusters
- High risk of substance abuse in attempt to alleviate anxiety

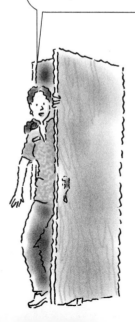

Many people with this disorder adopt a restricted lifestyle, including avoiding public places and new or unfamiliar settings, to prevent recurrence of a panic attack.

What causes it

- May stem from a combination of physical and psychological factors
- May have a hereditary component
- May develop from maladaptive learned behavior

What to look for

- Repeated episodes of unexpected apprehension, fear, and impending doom
- Lasts for minutes or hours; can be daily or intermittent
- During an attack
  - Hyperventilation, difficulty breathing, sensation of smothering, choking, or lump in throat
  - Tachycardia, palpitations
  - Trembling and weakness
  - Dizziness, tingling sensation or light-headedness
  - Fidgeting or pacing, desire to flee
  - Rapid speech
  - Profuse sweating
  - Digestive disturbances
  - Chest pain or pressure
  - Feelings of unreality or detachment from self
  - Fear of losing control or going crazy
  - Fear of dying
  - Chills or hot flashes
- Upset, fear, and exhaustion after the attack

This is intense

Managing an acute panic attack

If your patient experiences an acute panic attack, follow these guidelines:

• Maintain a calm, serene approach.
• Stay with the patient until the attack subsides.
• Assure the patient that you are in control of the immediate situation.
• Avoid insincere expressions of reassurance.
• Reduce stimuli such as bright lights and noise.
• Give the patient brief, simple directions, one at a time.
• Allow the patient to move around the room to help expend energy, if safety is not an issue.
• Show the patient how to take slow, deep breaths if he's hyperventilating, and reinforce relaxation techniques.
• Avoid touching the patient unless you've established rapport—he may be too stimulated or frightened to be reassured.
• Encourage the patient to express his feelings.
• Administer prescribed medications.

How it's treated

• Cognitive-behavioral therapy
• Psychotherapy
• Relaxation techniques
• Antianxiety drugs and antidepressants
• Beta-adrenergic blockers for symptomatic relief during an attack

Parkinson's disease

- Degenerative neurologic disease
- Characterized by dopamine deficiency that prevents affected brain cells from performing normal inhibitory functions in the CNS
- Produces progressive muscle rigidity, akinesia, and involuntary tremor

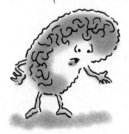

Lack of dopamine produces the progressive muscle rigidity, akinesis, and involuntary tremor characteristic of Parkinson's disease.

I see, I see

Neurotransmitter action in Parkinson's disease

Parkinson's disease is a degenerative process involving the dopaminergic neurons in the substantia nigra (the area of the basal ganglia that produces and stores the neurotransmitter dopamine). Dopamine deficiency prevents affected brain cells from performing their normal inhibitory function. Other nondopaminergic receptors may be affected, possibly contributing to depression and other nonmotor symptoms.

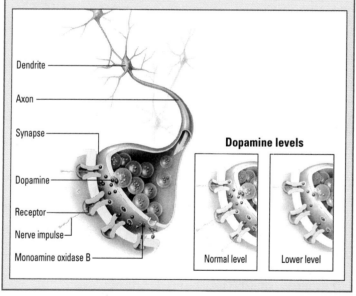

What causes it

- Exact cause unknown
- May be combination of genetic susceptibility and exposure to environmental stressors

- May result from exposure to toxins (manganese dust, carbon monoxide, pesticides, certain drugs)
- Increased incidence with repeated brain injury, including professional athletes

What to look for

- Muscle rigidity—resistance to passive muscle stretching
  - Uniform (lead-pipe rigidity)
  - Jerky (cogwheel rigidity)
- Bradykinesia causing difficulty walking; gait becomes shuffling
- Akinesia producing a high-pitched, monotone voice; drooling; masklike facial expression; stooped posture; and freezing movement, dysarthria, or dysphagia
- Insidious resting tremor that begins in the fingers (unilateral pill-roll tremor), increases during stress or anxiety, and decreases with purposeful movement and sleep
- Excessive sweating and oily skin
- Decreased motility of GI and GU smooth muscle
- Orthostatic hypotension

How it's treated

- Treatment aimed at symptom control
- Levodopa (which is converted to dopamine by the brain)
  - Most effective during early stages
  - Given in increasing doses until symptoms are relieved or adverse effects appear
  - Usually given with carbidopa, an enzyme inhibitor that slows the breakdown of levodopa by the body
- Dopamine agonists (may be used early in disease or in combination with levodopa) to enhance response or decrease adverse effects
- Alternative drug therapy (anticholinergics, antihistamines, amantadine, an antiviral or selegiline, an MAO inhibitor) when levodopa is ineffective, to conserve dopamine and enhance the therapeutic effect of levodopa

- Stereotactic neurosurgery to control involuntary movement by ablating selected areas of the brain
- Deep brain stimulation (alternative when conventional treatment fails) to decrease tremors and allow normal function
- Active and passive ROM exercises, daily activities, walking, and massage to help relax muscles
- Referral to National Parkinson Foundation or United Parkinson Foundation to provide information and support

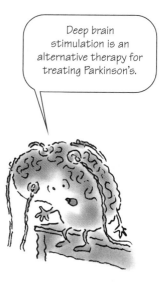

Polycystic ovarian syndrome

- Long-standing anovulation and excess of androgens (male hormones)
- Characterized by formation of 8 or more follicular cysts in the ovaries related to the failure to release an egg
- Long-term effects including diabetes, heart disease, and endometrial or breast cancer

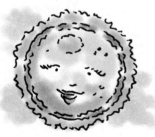

Excess androgens and the presence of multiple follicular cysts that fail to release an egg are characteristic of this disorder, which is a leading cause of infertility in females.

What causes it
- Unknown
- Possible genetic factor

What to look for
- Mild pelvic discomfort, lower back pain
- Dyspareunia
- Menstrual disturbance
- Abnormal uterine bleeding
- Hirsutism, acne, male-pattern hair loss
- Obesity
- Diabetes with insulin resistance
- Hypercholesterolemia
- Hypertension
- Infertility

How it's treated
- Clomiphene to induce ovulation
- Metformin for diabetes
- Medroxyprogesterone for infertility
- Low-dose hormonal contraceptives to treat abnormal bleeding in patients needing contraception
- Weight loss, diet, exercise, and stress reduction (obesity and stress can contribute to androgen excess)
- Symptomatic treatment of acne and hair loss with spironolactone and of hair loss with propecia
- Analgesics for pain relief
- Surgery if ovarian cyst is persistent or suspicious

Prostate cancer

- Slow-growing, most common neoplasm in men older than age 50
- Commonly forms as adenocarcinoma (derived from glandular tissue); sarcomas rarely occur
- Usually originates in posterior prostate gland; sometimes originates near urethra
- Seldom results from benign hyperplastic enlargement (which is common with aging)
- Clinical manifestations typically associated with later stages of disease

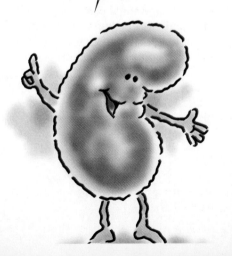

Even though prostate cancer is usually slow-growing, don't waste any time checking out unusual urinary symptoms.

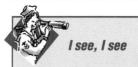

I see, I see

How prostate cancer develops

Prostate cancer grows slowly. When primary lesions metastasize beyond the prostate, they invade the prostate capsule and spread along the ejaculatory ducts in the space between the seminal vesicles.

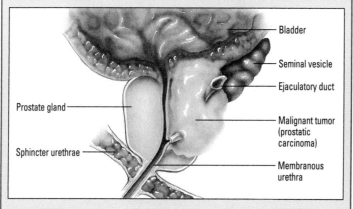

Bladder

Seminal vesicle

Ejaculatory duct

Prostate gland

Malignant tumor (prostatic carcinoma)

Sphincter urethrae

Membranous urethra

What causes it

- Exact cause unknown

Risk factors

- Race or ethnic origin (highest reported incidence in black men)
- Age (incidence rapidly increases after age 50)
- Genetic component (increased risk in men whose first-degree relative has prostate cancer)
- Exposure to environmental and occupational toxins
- Smoking and high-fat diet

What to look for

- Difficulty initiating urine stream
- Dribbling, urine retention, unexplained cystitis
- Back pain
- Pain with urination, ejaculation, and bowel movement
- Hematuria (rare)

How it's treated

- Radiation therapy to treat locally invasive lesions (may also relieve bone pain associated with metastasis)
- Radioactive seed implants into prostate (brachytherapy) to enhance radiation of cancerous area with minimal exposure to surrounding tissue
- Hormonal therapy (flutamide) to treat androgen-dependent prostate cancer
- Radical prostatectomy to remove prostate gland and tumor
- Transurethral resection of prostate to relieve obstruction
- Orchiectomy to decrease androgen production
- Cryoablation to remove tumor by freezing
- Chemotherapy as palliative treatment for metastatic prostate cancer
- Pain management to alleviate pain associated with bone metastasis
- Routine PSA testing to monitor treatment

Psoriasis

- Chronic, noncontagious skin disease characterized by epidermal proliferation with recurring partial remissions and exacerbations
- Flare-ups commonly related to specific systemic and environmental factors but may be unpredictable
- Exfoliative or erythrodermic psoriasis signifies widespread involvement

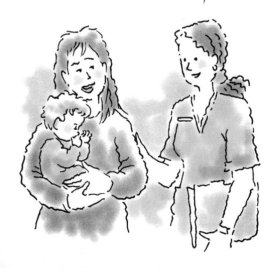

I see, I see

Understanding psoriasis

Psoriasis is a chronic, noncontagious, inflammatory skin disease marked by reddish papules (solid elevations) and plaques covered with silvery scales. Psoriatic skin cells have a shortened maturation time as they migrate from the basal membrane to the surface or stratum corneum. As a result, the stratum corneum develops thick, scaly silver plaques, the chief sign of psoriasis.

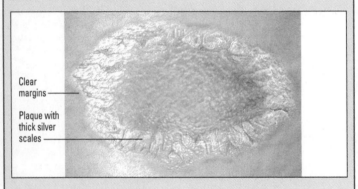

Clear margins —

Plaque with thick silver scales —

What causes it

- Genetic predisposition
- Drugs (lithium, beta-adrenergic blockers)
- Possible immune disorder (associated with presence of human leukocyte antigens)
- Environmental factors
- Isomorphic effect or Koebner's phenomenon (lesions develop at sites of injury due to trauma)
- Beta-hemolytic streptococcal infections (associated with certain flare-ups)
- Pregnancy

- Endocrine changes
- Climate (cold weather tends to exacerbate psoriasis)
- Emotional stress

What to look for

- Itching—and occasionally pain—from dry, cracked, encrusted lesions
- Erythematous and usually well-defined plaques, sometimes covering large areas of the body (psoriatic lesions)
- Lesions most commonly on scalp, chest, elbows, knees, back, face, soles, and palms
- Characteristic silver scales that either flake off easily or thicken, covering lesion
- Fine bleeding from scale removal
- Occasional appearance of small guttate lesions (usually thin and erythematous with few scales), either alone or with plaques
- Small indentations and yellow or brown discoloration of the nails
- Arthritic symptoms in finger, toe, or sacroiliac joints

How it's treated

- UVB or natural sunlight exposure to retard rapid cell production to point of minimal erythema
- Topical therapy (steroid creams and ointments, anthralin ointment, calcipotriene ointment, coal tar, tazarotene, salicylic acid) to control symptoms
- Goeckerman regimen (combines tar baths and UVB treatments) to help achieve remission and clear skin in 3 to 5 weeks (severe chronic psoriasis)
- Psoralens (plant extracts that accelerate exfoliation) with exposure to high-intensity UVA light (PUVA therapy) to retard rapid cell production
- TNF-blockers (etanercept, infliximab) to stop inflammation and quiet psoriasis

- Immunomodulators (alefacept, methotrexate, cyclosporine) to treat extensive, widespread, or resistant disease
- Retinoids (acitretin, tazarotene) to stimulate cell differentiation and inhibit malignant transformation in skin
- Low-dose antihistamines, oatmeal baths, emollients, hydrocolloid dressings, and open wet dressings to help relieve pruritus
- Referral to National Psoriasis Foundation for information and support

Pulmonary hypertension

- Increase in pulmonary artery pressure (PAP) above normal (mean PAP of 25 mm Hg or more) that occurs for reasons other than aging or altitude
- May be classified as primary (idiopathic) or secondary
  - Primary characterized by increased PAP and increased pulmonary vascular resistance (with no obvious cause); most common in women ages 20 to 40
  - Secondary resulting from existing cardiac or pulmonary disease (or both)

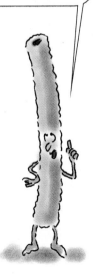

Regardless of the cause, pulmonary hypertension is serious business and, left untreated, eventually leads to right-sided heart failure.

I see, I see

Understanding pulmonary hypertension

In pulmonary hypertension, smooth muscle in the pulmonary artery wall hypertrophies for no known reason, narrowing the small pulmonary artery (arterioles) or obliterating it completely. Fibrous lesions also form around the vessels, impairing distensibility and increasing vascular resistance. Increased pressures generated in the lungs are transmitted to the right ventricle, which supplies the pulmonary artery. Eventually, the right ventricle fails.

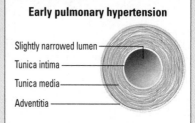

Early pulmonary hypertension

Slightly narrowed lumen

Tunica intima

Tunica media

Adventitia

Late pulmonary hypertension

Critically narrowed lumen

Tunica intima

Tunica media

Adventitia

What causes it

- Primary: possibly hereditary factors or altered immune mechanisms
- Secondary: diseases such as COPD, diffuse interstitial pneumonia, malignant metastasis, scleroderma, obesity, pulmonary embolism, vasculitis, rheumatic valvular disease, mitral stenosis, ventricular septal defect, and left-sided heart failure

What to look for

- Dyspnea on exertion, shortness of breath, pain with breathing
- Decreased diaphragmatic excursion and decreased or loud tubular breath sounds
- Hypotension, tachycardia
- Fatigue, weakness
- Syncope
- Ascites, jugular vein distention, peripheral edema from right-sided heart failure
- Easily palpable right ventricular lift, displaced PMI
- Systolic ejection murmur; split S_2, S_3, and S_4
- Reduced carotid pulse

How it's treated

- Oxygen therapy to correct hypoxemia and resulting increased pulmonary vascular resistance
- Fluid restriction (in right-sided heart failure) to decrease heart's workload
- Digoxin to increase cardiac output
- Diuretics to decrease intravascular volume and extravascular fluid accumulation
- Vasodilators to reduce myocardial workload and oxygen consumption
- Calcium channel blockers to reduce myocardial workload and oxygen consumption

- Bronchodilators to relax smooth muscles and increase air-way patency
- Beta-adrenergic blockers to improve oxygenation
- Treatment of underlying cause to correct pulmonary edema
- Heart-lung transplant to treat severe cases

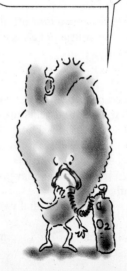

Various treatments for pulmonary hypertension focus on ways to reduce myocardial workload and oxygen consumption.

Renal failure, chronic

- Usually end result of gradual tissue destruction and loss of renal function
- May also result from rapidly progressing disease of sudden onset that destroys nephrons and causes irreversible kidney damage
- Few symptoms until less than 25% of glomerular filtration remains; normal parenchyma then deteriorates rapidly, and symptoms worsen as renal function decreases
- Fatal without treatment; dialysis or kidney transplant can sustain life

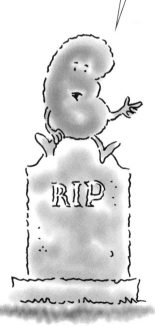

Without treatment, chronic renal failure spells "The end."

I see, I see

Understanding chronic renal failure

Decreasing number of functioning nephrons

▼

Increased solute load per nephron

▼

Alteration in GFR

▼

Reduced renal reserve
GFR of 35% to 50% of normal
No signs of impaired renal function

▼

Renal insufficiency
GFR of 20% to 35% of normal
Possible hypertension, azotemia, and anemia

▼

Renal failure
GFR of 20% to 25% of normal
Uremia; neurologic, cardiovascular, and GI symptoms

▼

End-stage renal disease
GFR less than 20% of normal
Atrophy and fibrosis in renal tubules

What causes it

- Diabetes
- Hypertension
- Chronic glomerular disease (glomerulonephritis)
- Nephrotoxic agents or chronic infection
- Congenital anomalies (polycystic kidney disease)
- Vascular collagen or endocrine disease

- Obstruction (renal calculi)
- Collagen disease (SLE)

What to look for

- Fluid and electrolyte imbalances
  - Hypervolemia
  - Hypocalcemia
  - Hyperkalemia
  - Hyperphosphatemia
  - Metabolic acidosis
- Edema
- Dry mouth, nausea
- Fatigue, altered mental state
- Irregular heart rate, cardiac irritability
- Hypertension
- Muscle cramps and twitching
- Kussmaul's respirations
- Bone and muscle pain, fractures
- Peripheral neuropathy
- Yellow-bronze skin, dry scaly skin; severe itching
- Azotemia
- GI bleeding, hemorrhage, bruising; gum soreness and bleeding from anemia, thrombocytopenia, and platelet defects
- Susceptibility to infection

How it's treated

- Low-protein diet to limit accumulation of end products of protein metabolism that kidneys can't excrete
- Sodium, potassium, and fluid restrictions to maintain fluid and electrolyte balance
- Loop diuretics (furosemide) to maintain fluid balance
- Cardiac glycosides (digoxin) to mobilize fluids causing edema (monitor carefully for toxicity)
- Calcium carbonate or calcium acetate to treat renal osteodystrophy by binding phosphate and supplementing calcium
- Calcitrol to treat hypocalcemia

- Antihypertensives (ACE inhibitors) to control blood pressure and edema
- Famotidine or ranitidine to decrease gastric irritation
- Iron and folate supplements or RBC transfusion for anemia
- Synthetic erythropoietin to stimulate bone marrow to produce RBCs
- Supplemental iron, conjugated estrogens, and desmopressin to combat hematologic effects
- Peritoneal dialysis or hemodialysis to treat fluid imbalance and help control end-stage renal disease
- Renal transplantation (usually treatment of choice if donor is available) to replace patient's malfunctioning kidneys

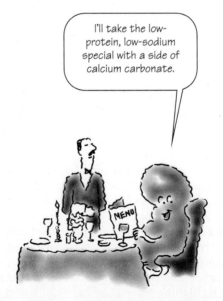

Rheumatoid arthritis

- Chronic, systemic autoimmune inflammatory disease of connective tissue that attacks primarily peripheral joints and surrounding muscles, tendons, ligaments, and blood vessels
- Involves partial remissions and unpredictable exacerbations

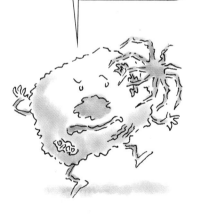

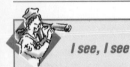

I see, I see

Understanding rheumatoid arthritis

If not arrested, the inflammatory process occurs in four stages:
1. Synovitis develops from congestion and edema of the synovial membrane and joint capsule. Infiltration by lymphocytes, macrophages, and neutrophils continues the local inflammatory response. These cells, as well as fibroblast-like synovial cells, produce enzymes that help degrade bone and cartilage.
2. Pannus (thickened layers of granulation tissue) covers and invades cartilage, eventually destroying the joint capsule and bone.
3. Fibrous ankylosis (fibrous invasion of the pannus and scar formation) occludes the joint space. Bone atrophy and misalignment cause visible deformities and disrupt the articulation of opposing bones, causing muscle atrophy and imbalance and, possibly, partial dislocations.
4. Fibrous tissue calcifies, causing bony ankylosis and total immobility.

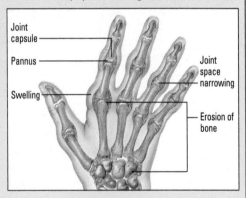

What causes it
- Unknown
- May have genetic, infectious, and endocrine factors

What to look for

- Usually develops insidiously with nonspecific signs and symptoms
  - Fatigue, malaise
  - Anorexia
  - Persistent low-grade fever
  - Weight loss
  - Lymphadenopathy
  - Vague articular joint symptoms
- Joint stiffness after inactivity, especially in the morning
- Spindle shape of the fingers from edema and joint congestion and flexion deformities
- Tender, painful joints, at first only with movement, eventually at rest
- Loss of joint function
- Joint hot to the touch
- Carpal tunnel syndrome
- Appearance of rheumatoid nodules—subcutaneous, round or oval, nontender masses, usually on pressure areas such as elbows
- Vasculitis, which can lead to skin lesions, leg ulcers, and multiple systemic complications
- Pericardial and pleural effusions
- Anemia

How it's treated

- DMARDs (disease-modifying anti-rheumatic drugs)
  - Antimalarials (hydroxychloroquine sulfate), sulfasalazine, gold salts, and D-penicillamine to reduce acute and chronic inflammation
  - Azathioprine, cyclosporine, or methotrexate for immunosuppression in early disease (suppresses T- and B-lymphocyte proliferation, which destroys synovium)

- Biologic response modifiers, such as infliximab, adalimumab, and etanercept, to block the inflammatory response that leads to joint damage
- Nonsteroidal anti-inflammatory drugs (NSAIDs), such as fenoprofen, ibuprofen, and indomethacin, to relieve inflammation and pain, including second generation NSAIDS, the COX-2 inhibitors that are under monitored use (celecoxib)
- Corticosteroids (prednisone) for anti-inflammatory effects (low doses); higher doses for immunosuppressive effect on T-cells
- Salicylates, to decrease inflammation and relieve joint pain
- Analgesics for pain control
- Synovectomy (removal of destructive, proliferating synovium, usually in wrists, knees, and fingers) to possibly halt or delay disease course
- Osteotomy (cutting of bone or excision of bone wedge) to realign joint surfaces and redistribute stress
- Tendon transfers to prevent deformities or relieve contractures
- Joint reconstruction or total joint arthroplasty (including metatarsal head and distal ulnar resectional arthroplasty, insertion of a Silastic prosthesis between metacarpophalangeal and proximal interphalangeal joints) to treat and correct deformities in severe disease
- Arthrodesis (joint fusion) for stability and pain relief (sacrifices joint mobility)
- Supportive measures, such as adequate rest, splinting affected joints, physical therapy, heat or ice application

Sarcoidosis

- Multisystem, granulomatous disorder
- Produces lymphadenopathy, pulmonary infiltration, and skeletal, liver, eye, or skin lesions
- Symptoms lasting from a couple of years to end of life and varying by extent and location of fibrosis
- Pulmonary fibrosis and pulmonary disability associated with chronic, progressive type

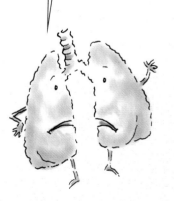

I see, I see

Understanding lung changes in sarcoidosis

Excessive inflammatory response starts in the alveoli, bronchioles, and blood vessels of the lungs. Fibroblasts, mast cells, collagen fibers, and proteoglycans encase the inflammatory and immune cells, creating granulomas. Organ dysfunction results when granulomas accumulate, distorting the normal tissue architecture and causing alveolitis and scarring.

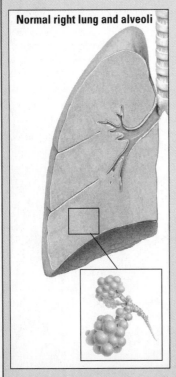

Normal right lung and alveoli

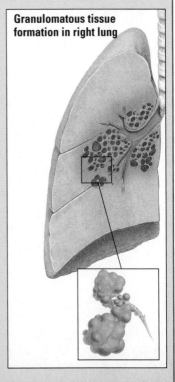

Granulomatous tissue formation in right lung

What causes it

- Unknown
- Possible related factors
  - Hypersensitivity response or extreme immune response
  - Genetic predisposition
  - Chemical exposure

What to look for

- Initially, arthralgia of the wrists, ankles, and elbows; fatigue, malaise; weight loss
- Breathlessness, cough, substernal pain
- Pulmonary hypertension and cor pulmonale in advanced cases
- Skin and nasal mucosal lesions
- Anterior uveitis, glaucoma, and (rarely) blindness
- Muscle weakness, polyarthralgia
- Arrhythmias
- Lymphadenopathy and splenomegaly
- Cranial or peripheral nerve palsies, basilar meningitis, seizures
- Diabetes insipidus from pituitary and hypothalamic lesions
- Hypercalcemia

How it's treated

- Corticosteroids to reduce inflammation and resulting damage
- Antimalarial drugs (hydroxychloroquine, chloroquine) for anti-inflammatory effects
- Immunosuppressive agents (methotrexate, azathioprine) to decrease immune response
- Organ-specific treatment for heart or respiratory failure, arrhythmias, and other symptoms
- Transplantation if organ failure occurs
- Low-calcium diet and avoidance of sunlight exposure

Schizophrenia

- Group of severe, disabling psychiatric disorders
- Marked by withdrawal from reality, illogical thinking, possible delusions and hallucinations, and other emotional, behavioral, or intellectual disturbances
- May alter speech, affect, and perception, psychomotor behavior, interpersonal skills, and sense of self
- Presence of prodromal or residual symptoms in addition to at least 1 month of active symptoms during a minimum 6-month period
- Recognized types:
  - Paranoid
  - Disorganized
  - Catatonic
  - Undifferentiated
  - Residual

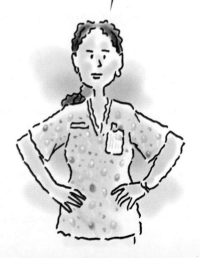

Expect to note marked withdrawal from reality, illogical thinking, and other emotional, behavioral, and intellectual disturbances in someone with schizophrenia.

What causes it
- Unknown
- May result from combination of genetic, biological, cultural, and psychological factors

What to look for
- Variety of abnormal behaviors related to disorder
- Two or more of the following symptoms present for a significant time during a 1-month period unless treated
  - Delusions
  - Hallucinations, including hearing voices
  - Disorganized speech
  - Grossly disorganized or catatonic behavior
  - Negative symptoms (flat affect, inability to speak, anhedonia, attention impairment, apathy, and avolition)
- Social and occupational dysfunction
- Exclusion of other psychiatric or medical disorders or cause by a substance

How it's treated
- Antipsychotic, antidepressant, and anxiolytic drugs to control symptoms
- Psychotherapy in addition to other treatments to provide emotional support and positive reinforcement
- Psychosocial rehabilitation, education, and social skills training based on patient's level of impaired functioning
- Family therapy
- Electroconvulsive therapy (ECT) for acute treatment and for those intolerant of or unresponsive to medication

Scleroderma

- Also known as progressive systemic sclerosis
- Diffuse connective tissue disease
- Occurs in several distinctive forms, including CREST syndrome, localized scleroderma, and graft-versus-host disease
- Symptoms based on systems affected

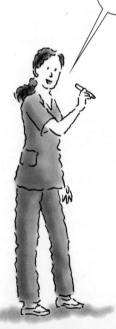

CREST syndrome is a limited form of scleroderma characterized by calcinosis, Raynaud's phenomenon, esophageal dysfunction, sclerodactyly, and telangiectasia.

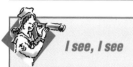

I see, I see

How scleroderma develops

Scleroderma is an uncommon connective tissue disorder marked by inflammatory, degenerative, and fibrotic changes of many body organs.

Degenerative and fibrotic changes in skin, blood vessels, synovial membranes, skeletal muscles, and internal organs (especially the esophagus, intestinal tract, thyroid, heart, lungs, and kidneys) follow initial inflammation.

Disease usually begins in fingers and extends to upper arms, shoulders, neck, and face.

Skin begins to atrophy.

Edema and infiltrates containing CD4+ T cells surround blood vessels.

Inflamed collagen fibers begin to degenerate and become edematous, losing strength and elasticity.

Dermis becomes tightly bound to underlying structures.

Affected dermal appendages atrophy; osteoporosis destroys distal phalanges.

As disease progresses, fibrosis and atrophy can affect other areas, including muscles and joints.

What causes it

- Unknown
- Risk factors
  - Exposure to silica dust and polyvinyl chloride
  - Anticancer agents such as bleomycin
  - Nonopioid analgesics such as pentazocine
  - Viral infections

What to look for

- Raynaud's phenomenon
- Progressive phalangeal resorption, shortening fingers
- Pain, stiffness, and finger and joint swelling
- Skin thickening, producing taut, shiny skin over the entire hand and forearm
- Tight, inelastic facial skin, causing a masklike appearance and pinching of the mouth
- Slow-healing ulcerations on the fingertips or toes leading to gangrene
- GI dysfunction
  - Frequent reflux, heartburn
  - Dysphagia
  - Bloating after meals, abdominal distention
  - Diarrhea
  - Constipation
  - Malodorous floating stools
  - Weight loss
- Hypertension
- Arrhythmias
- Renal or respiratory failure

How it's treated

- Immunosuppressants to decrease immune response
- Corticosteroids and cochicine to stabilize symptoms
- Supportive care of ulcerations on digits, including surgical debridement if needed

- Calcium channel blockers, angiotensin II receptor antagonists or angiotensin-converting enzyme inhibitors, and low-dose coated aspirin for Raynaud's phenomenon
- Antacids, H_2 blockers, or proton pump inhibitors for reflux
- Periodic esophageal dilation and a soft, bland diet for esophagitis with stricture
- NSAIDs for pain relief
- Supportive treatment of symptoms from other systems involved

Scoliosis

- Lateral curvature of the spine
- May be thoracic, lumbar, or thoracolumbar
- May cause rib cage deformity

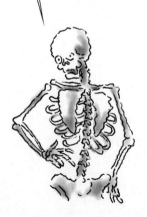

What causes it

- Functional (postural)
  - Usually results from discrepancy in leg lengths
- Structural
  - Congenital deformity
  - Paralytic or musculoskeletal; develops several months after asymmetrical paralysis of the trunk muscles (polio, cerebral palsy, muscular dystrophy)
  - Idiopathic (most common); appears during growth years and is caused by equilibrium dysfunction, familial tendency, or asymmetrical growth

What to look for

- Spinal curvature, most commonly to the right, with compensatory curve above or below
- Asymmetrical musculature
- Kyphosis (roundback) or lordosis (swayback)
- Backache
- Fatigue
- Dyspnea

How it's treated

- Spinal bracing
- Exercise with and without brace
- Spinal fusion and internal stabilization for progression despite bracing

Sickle cell anemia

- Congenital hemolytic anemia resulting from defective hemoglobin molecules (hemoglobin S); produces characteristic sickle-shaped red blood cells (RBCs)
- Occurs primarily in those of African and Mediterranean descent
- Symptoms typically appear after age 6 months (due to presence of large amount of fetal hemoglobin)

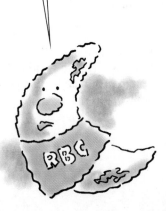

My unusual shape causes cells to clump together and stick to capillary walls during a crisis, blocking blood flow and causing cellular hypoxia.

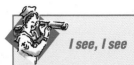

I see, I see

Understanding sickle cell crisis

Infection, exposure to cold, high altitudes, overexertion, or other situations that cause cellular oxygen deprivation may trigger a sickle cell crisis. The oxygenated, sickle-shaped RBCs stick to the capillary wall and each other, blocking blood flow and causing cellular hypoxia. The crisis worsens as tissue hypoxia and acidic waste products cause more sickling and cell damage. With each new crisis, organs and tissues (especially the kidneys and spleen) are slowly destroyed.

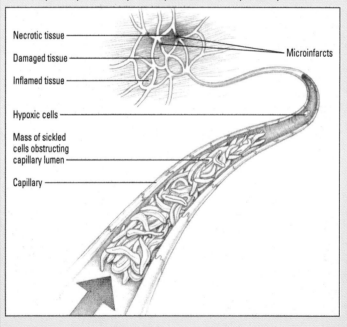

Necrotic tissue

Damaged tissue

Inflamed tissue

Microinfarcts

Hypoxic cells

Mass of sickled cells obstructing capillary lumen

Capillary

What causes it

- Autosomal recessive inheritance (homozygous inheritance of hemoglobin S-producing gene)

What to look for

- Tachycardia, cardiomegaly
- Chronic fatigue, lethargy, listlessness, sleepiness
- Unexplained dyspnea
- Hepatomegaly
- Joint swelling and pain, aching bones, pain in muscles
- Pale lips, tongue, palms, or nail beds
- Jaundice
- Irritability
- Fever
- Susceptibility to infection

How it's treated

- In acute episode, copious amounts of oral or I.V. fluids to correct hypovolemia and prevent dehydration and vessel occlusion
- Packed RBC transfusion to correct anemia or hypovolemia (if hemoglobin levels decrease)
- Sedation and analgesics for pain
- Oxygen administration to correct hypoxia
- Ventilatory assistance for respiratory failure
- Hydroxyurea to reduce painful episodes by increasing production of fetal hemoglobin
- Iron and folic acid supplements to prevent megaloblastic anemia
- Prophylactic penicillin (after age 2 months) to prevent infection
- Bone marrow transplantation

Sjögren's syndrome

- Autoimmune rheumatic disorder
- Typically seen as diminished lacrimal and salivary gland secretion due to damage from lymphocytic infiltration
- May be primary or associated with connective tissue disorders, such as rheumatoid arthritis, scleroderma, and systemic lupus erythematosus
- May be limited to exocrine glands or involve other organs, such as the lungs and kidneys

What causes it
- Unknown
- May involve genetic and environmental factors

What to look for
- Severe dryness of the eyes
  - Foreign body sensation
  - Redness, burning, itching
  - Photosensitivity
  - Eye fatigue
  - Mucoid discharge and sensation of film across visual field
- Severe oral dryness
  - Difficulty swallowing and talking
  - Abnormal taste or smell
  - Thirst
  - Ulcers of the tongue, buccal mucosa, and lips
  - Severe dental caries
- Dryness of other mucosa
  - Epistaxis
  - Hoarseness, nonproductive cough
  - Recurrent otitis media and respiratory infections
- Generalized itching
- Palpable purpura from vasculitis, especially on legs
- Recurrent low-grade fever
- Arthralgia or myalgia
- Hypothyroidism
- Lymph node enlargement
- Raynaud's phenomenon

How it's treated
- Moistening mouth and drinking plenty of fluids
- Meticulous oral hygiene
- Artificial tear and saliva preparations
- Eye ointment
- Salivation-stimulating medications (pilocarpine)

- Antibiotics or antifungals to treat infection
- Local heat and analgesics for discomfort
- Corticosteroids or immunosuppressants for pulmonary and renal interstitial disease
- Chemotherapy, surgery, or radiation to treat accompanying lymphoma (rare)

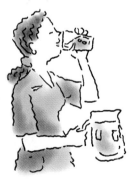

Drinking plenty of fluids and using artificial tears and saliva preparations can help manage some of the persistent symptoms of this autoimmune disease.

Spinal cord injury

- Complete injury—total lack of sensory and motor function below the level of injury
- Incomplete injury—some sensory or motor function below the injury
- Signs and symptoms dependent on level and severity of injury
- Incidence highest in males between age 15 and 35

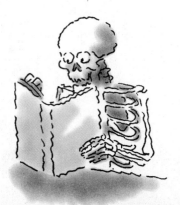

Says here 'Depending on the level and severity of injury, symptoms can range from pain and loss of sensation or movement to difficulty breathing, coughing, and clearing secretions.' Now that's nothing to sneeze at!

I see, I see

What happens in spinal cord injury

Injury causes inflammatory process.

Ensuing edema causes compression and decreased blood supply.

Edema temporarily adds to the patient's dysfunction by increasing pressure and compressing the nerves.

Phagocytes appear at the site within 36 to 48 hours after the injury, macrophages engulf the degenerating axons, and collagen replaces normal tissue.

Scarring and meningeal thickening leave the nerves in the area blocked or tangled, causing permanent deficits.

What causes it

- Traumatic injury that fractures or dislocates vertebrae, displacing bone fragments, disc material, or ligaments and causing bruising or tearing of the spinal cord tissue
- Nontraumatic events, including arthritis; cancer; ischemia, bleeding, infection, or inflammation of the spinal cord; or disc degeneration

What to look for

- Pain or intense stinging caused by damage to nerve fibers in the spinal cord
- Loss of movement
- Loss of sensation, including the ability to feel heat, cold, and touch

- Loss of bowel or bladder control
- Exaggerated reflex activities or spasms
- Changes in sexual function, sexual sensitivity, and fertility
- Difficulty breathing, coughing, or clearing secretions from the lungs

How it's treated

- Rehabilitation programs—physical and occupational therapy, assistive devices to maximize independence
- Respiratory support and prevention of respiratory complications
- Prevention of complications of immobility, such as deconditioning, blood clots, bed sores, muscle contractions, and urinary tract infections
- Pain control
- Bowel and bladder training or management
- Social and emotional support
- Nutritional support for healthy diet and weight control

Squamous cell carcinoma

- Invasive tumor with metastatic potential that arises from keratinizing epidermal cells
- Occurs most commonly in fair-skinned white men older than age 60
- Higher incidence with outdoor employment or recreation or residence in a sunny, warm climate

I see, I see

How squamous cell carcinoma develops

Squamous cell carcinoma is an invasive tumor with metastatic potential that arises from the keratinizing epidermal cells. It begins as a firm red nodule or scaly, crusted, flat lesion that may remain confined to the epidermis for a period of time. It eventually spreads to the dermis; untreated, it will spread to regional lymph nodes.

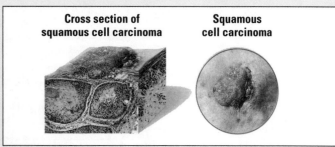

Cross section of squamous cell carcinoma

Squamous cell carcinoma

What causes it

- Common predisposing factors
  - Overexposure to sun's UV rays
  - Presence of premalignant lesions
- X-ray therapy
- Ingestion of herbicides containing arsenic
- Chronic skin irritation and inflammation, burns, or scars
- Exposure to local carcinogens (tar, oil)
- Hereditary diseases (xeroderma pigmentosum, albinism)
- Site of smallpox vaccination, psoriasis, or chronic discoid lupus erythematosus (rare)

What to look for

- Nodule with firm, indurated base

- Scaling and ulceration of opaque, firm nodules with indistinct borders
- Commonly on face, ear, dorsa of hand and forearm or other sun-damaged areas
- Systemic metastatic symptoms of pain, malaise, fatigue, weakness, anorexia

How it's treated

- Wide surgical excision to remove lesion
- Mohs micrographic surgery—highest cure rate
- Electrodesiccation and curettage to remove lesion (offer good cosmetic results for small lesions)
- Cryosurgery for smaller, nonfacial lesions
- Radiation therapy (generally for elderly or debilitated patients and recurrent lesions)
- Chemosurgery (reserved for resistant or recurrent lesions)
- Lymph node removal depending on location of lesion to node
- Skin grafting and reconstructive surgery
- Systemic chemotherapy for carcinoma with metastasis
- Avoidance of excessive sun exposure, wearing protective clothing, and using sunscreen (containing para-aminobenzoic acid, benzophenone, and zinc) and lip balm to minimize risk of future sun damage
- Regular screening and follow-up

Stroke

- Sudden impairment of cerebral circulation in one or more blood vessels
- Varying symptoms according to affected artery, severity of damage, and extent of collateral circulation
- Stroke in one hemisphere, which causes features on opposite side
- Stroke that damages cranial nerves and affects structures on same side
- Prompt identification of ischemic versus hemorrhagic stroke (crucial to guide treatment)

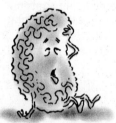

Stroke in one hemisphere of the brain causes changes and deficits on the opposite side...what a muddle!

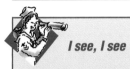

I see, I see

Understanding stroke

Strokes are typically classified as hemorrhagic or ischemic, depending on the underlying cause. In either type of stroke, the patient is deprived of oxygen and nutrients.

Hemorrhagic stroke
Hemorrhagic stroke is caused by bleeding within and around the brain. The bleeding that fills the spaces between the brain and the skull (called *subarachnoid hemorrhage*) is caused by ruptured aneurysms, arteriovenous malformation, and head trauma. Bleeding within the brain tissue itself (known as *intracerebral hemorrhage*) is primarily caused by hypertension.

Hemorrhagic stroke

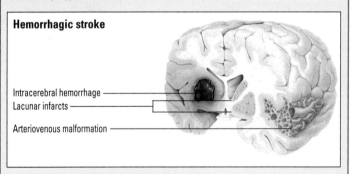

Intracerebral hemorrhage
Lacunar infarcts
Arteriovenous malformation

(continued)

Understanding stroke *(continued)*

Ischemic stroke

Ischemic stroke results from a blockage or reduction of blood flow to an area of the brain. The blockage may result from atherosclerosis (plaque formation) or blood clot (thrombus) formation.

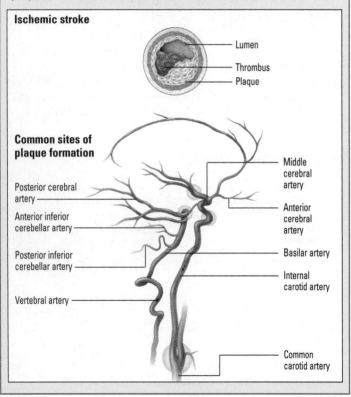

Ischemic stroke

- Lumen
- Thrombus
- Plaque

Common sites of plaque formation

- Middle cerebral artery
- Posterior cerebral artery
- Anterior cerebral artery
- Anterior inferior cerebellar artery
- Posterior inferior cerebellar artery
- Basilar artery
- Internal carotid artery
- Vertebral artery
- Common carotid artery

What causes it

- Spontaneous bleeding in brain (hemorrhagic stroke)
- Thrombosis or emboli (ischemic stroke)

Risk factors

- Hypertension, cardiac disease
- Family history of stroke
- History of transient ischemic attacks
- Diabetes, hyperlipidemia
- Cigarette smoking, increased alcohol intake
- Obesity, sedentary lifestyle
- Use of hormonal contraceptives
- Valvular disease or replacement
- Blood clotting disorders

What to look for

- Findings depend on artery affected

What happens in stroke

Artery affected	Signs and symptoms
Middle cerebral artery	Aphasia or dysphasia; visual field deficits; hemiparesis of affected side (more severe in face, arm)
Carotid artery	Weakness, paralysis, numbness; sensory changes; altered level of consciousness; bruits over carotid artery; headaches
Vertebrobasilar artery	Weakness, paralysis; numbness around lips and mouth; visual field deficits, diplopia, and nystagmus; poor coordination and dizziness; dysphagia, slurred speech; amnesia; ataxia
Anterior cerebral artery	Confusion; weakness, numbness; urinary incontinence; impaired motor and sensory functions; personality changes
Posterior cerebral artery	Visual field deficits; sensory impairment; dyslexia; cortical blindness; coma

How it's treated

- Rehabilitation therapy, including speech, physical, and occupational therapy
- Assistive devices to help maintain independence
- Anticoagulant therapy (heparin, warfarin) to maintain vessel patency and prevent further clot formation (initiated 24 hours after thrombolytic therapy) in ischemic stroke
- Beta-adrenergic blockers or other anti-hypertensives as indicated to manage blood pressure
- Antiplatelet agents (such as aspirin)
- Smoking cessation
- Cholesterol management

This is intense

Managing acute stroke

If your patient suffers an acute stroke, expect to follow these initial treatment guidelines:
• Assist with endotracheal intubation and mechanical ventilation, if needed, to provide adequate airway.
• Administer I.V. fluid therapy with normal saline or lactated Ringer's solution to maintain hydration.
• Frequently assess vital signs and neurologic status.
• Monitor ICP and administer osmotic diuretics (mannitol) to prevent further cerebral damage; elevate head of bed 20 to 30 degrees.
• Administer stool softeners to prevent straining, which increases ICP.
• Administer acetaminophen to treat fever.
• Administer anticonvulsants to treat or prevent seizures.

For hemorrhagic stroke
• Administer analgesics to relieve headache.
• Administer antihypertensive agents (labetalol, nitroprusside) to control blood pressure when systolic reading is greater than 200 mm Hg or diastolic reading is greater than 100 mm Hg.

For ischemic stroke
• Administer thrombolytic therapy (tissue plasminogen activator, alteplase) within first 3 hours after onset of symptoms to dissolve clot, remove occlusion, and restore blood flow, minimizing cerebral damage (unless contraindicated).

Thalassemia

- Hereditary group of hemolytic anemias
- Beta-thalassemia (most common type) occurs as major, intermedia, and minor

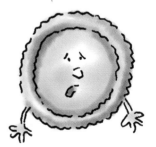

Reduced protein synthesis causes abnormal hemoglobin molecules, which in turn causes anemia, the presenting symptom of thalassemia.

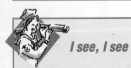

I see, I see

Understanding thalassemia

Thalassemia is characterized by defective synthesis in the polypeptide chains of hemoglobin's protein component; RBC synthesis is impaired. In thalassemia major, survival to adulthood seldom occurs. In thalassemia minor, a normal life span is expected. Severity depends on whether the patient is homozygous or heterozygous for the thalassemic trait.

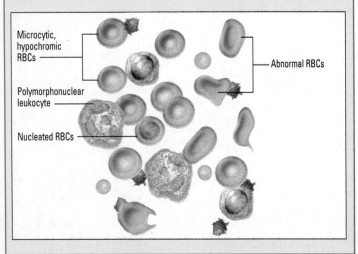

What causes it

- Homozygous inheritance of partially dominant autosomal gene (thalassemia major or intermedia)
- Heterozygous inheritance of the same gene (thalassemia minor)

What to look for

- Thalassemia major
  - Severe anemia
  - Bone abnormalities; children susceptible to pathologic fractures due to thinning of the long bones and expansion of the marrow cavities
  - Failure to thrive, anorexia
  - Pallor and jaundiced skin and sclera
  - Splenomegaly or hepatomegaly, with abdominal enlargement
  - Frequent infections
  - Bleeding tendencies
  - Small body and large head: may have mental retardation
- Thalassemia minor
  - Mild anemia

How it's treated

Thalassemia major

- Transfusions (packed RBCs) to increase hemoglobin levels
- Prompt treatment with appropriate antibiotics for infections
- Chelation therapy to remove excess iron from frequent blood transfusions
- Bone marrow transplantation (curative in some patients)

Thalassemia minor

- Patient teaching (condition is hereditary and may be mistaken for iron deficiency anemia)
- Genetic counseling (for adults desiring children)

Trigeminal neuralgia

- Painful disorder of the fifth cranial or trigeminal nerve
- Produces paroxysmal attacks of excruciating facial pain precipitated by stimulation of a trigger zone
- Can subside spontaneously and have long periods of remission

Lightly touching a trigger zone area, such as when applying make-up, can initiate a painful attack in someone with trigeminal neuralgia.

Trigeminal nerve function and distribution

Function
- Motor: chewing movements
- Sensory: sensations of face, scalp, and teeth (mouth and nasal chamber)

Distribution
I Ophthalmic
II Maxillary
III Mandibular

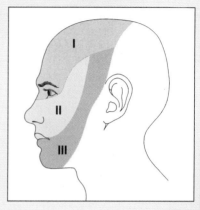

What causes it

- Believed to be related to a blood vessel pressing on the trigeminal nerve near the brain stem, resulting in nerve irritation
- Also associated with other disorders, such as multiple sclerosis, herpes zoster, and tumors that irritate or damage the myelin sheath
- May have a familial component

What to look for

- Reports of searing or burning pain, like an electric shock that lasts several seconds to 2 minutes in an area innervated by one of the divisions of the trigeminal nerve, least commonly the ophthalmic distribution
- Usually unilateral
- Attack initiated by light touch of the trigger zone
- Triggers: draft of air, exposure to heat or cold, eating or drinking, smiling, talking, applying make-up

- Patient's holding his face immobile to avoid an attack

How it's treated

- Anticonvulsants (carbamazepine, gabapentin) to relieve or prevent pain
- Antidepressants to relieve pain
- Percutaneous electrocoagulation of nerve rootlets
- Percutaneous radiofrequency ablation to destroy nerve root and relieve pain
- Microsurgery for vascular decompression
- Complementary and alternative medicine such as acupuncture, meditation, and hypnosis

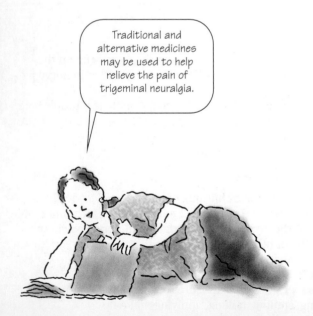

Traditional and alternative medicines may be used to help relieve the pain of trigeminal neuralgia.

Ulcerative colitis

- Inflammatory disease of the colon mucosa
- Begins in the rectum and sigmoid colon and extends upward; rarely affects the small intestine
- Produces edema and ulcerations
- Primarily affects young adults, especially women

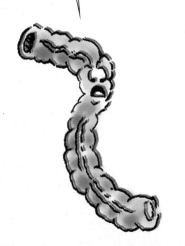

Ulcerative colitis causes recurrent attacks of bloody diarrhea—as many as 15 to 20 stools daily—which, as you can guess, makes me quite irritable.

What causes it

- Unknown
- May be an abnormal immune response to food or bacteria, such as *Escherichia coli*
- May have familial tendency

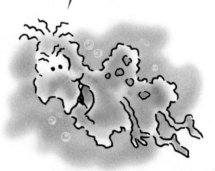

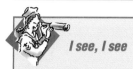

I see, I see

Understanding ulcerative colitis

Ulcerative colitis usually begins as inflammation in the base of the mucosal layer of the large intestine, developing into erosions that combine to form ulcers. The mucosa becomes diffusely ulcerated, leading to hemorrhage, edema, and exudate. Abscesses drain purulent material, become necrotic, and ulcerate further. Sloughing causes bloody, mucus-filled stools. As abscesses heal, scarring and thickening may appear in the bowel's inner muscle layer. Granulation tissue replaces the muscle layer and the colon narrows, shortens, and loses its characteristic folds.

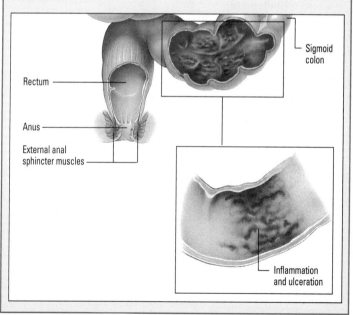

Sigmoid colon

Rectum

Anus

External anal sphincter muscles

Inflammation and ulceration

What to look for
- Recurrent attacks of bloody diarrhea, often containing pus and mucus
- As many as 15 to 20 stools daily
- Periods of asymptomatic remission
- Spastic rectum and anus
- Abdominal pain
- Irritability
- Weight loss, anorexia, nausea and vomiting

How it's treated
- Supportive treatment of acute episodes
  - Bed rest
  - Fluid replacement
  - Clear-liquid diet or TPN
- Blood transfusion or iron supplements to correct anemia
- Immunomodulators or 5-aminosalicylates to decrease the frequency of attack
- Corticosteroids to control inflammation
- Antispasmodics and antidiarrheals when colitis is under control but frequent, loose stools persist
- Antibiotics, as necessary
- Surgical resection as a last resort for toxic megacolon, failure to respond to treatment, or unbearable symptoms
- Routine monitoring for colon cancer

Urinary incontinence

- Uncontrolled passage of urine
- May involve large volumes of urine or scant dribbling
- Four types—stress, overflow, urge, and total

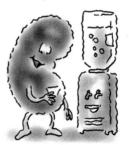

In many cases, it's not the volume of urine but the loss of bladder control or muscle tone that produces urinary incontinence.

What causes it

- Results from a wide range of conditions
- Weakened pelvic floor due to pregnancy and childbirth, pelvic trauma, or hormonal changes of menopause
- Urologic disorders, such as benign prostatic hyperplasia, bladder calculi, chronic prostatitis, urethral stricture, procedural damage to the urethral sphincter, bladder or prostate cancer
- Neurologic disorders, such as stroke, diabetic neuropathy, multiple sclerosis, spinal cord injury, dementias
- Drugs, such as diuretics, sedatives, hypnotics, antipsychotics, anticholinergics, and alpha-adrenergic blockers
- Caffeine

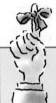

Memory jogger

The mnemonic **OUTS** helps you remember the main forms of urinary incontinence.

O: Overflow incontinence—urine loss occurring when a specific bladder volume is reached

U: Urge incontinence—urine loss from a bladder contraction that follows a strong, sudden need to urinate

T: Total incontinence—complete loss of urinary control, as from a non-functioning urethral sphincter muscle

S: Stress incontinence—loss of small amounts of urine (less than 50 ml) when abdominal pressure increases, such as when a person coughs, sneezes, or lifts a heavy object

What to look for

- Bladder distention
- Abnormal urination patterns
  - Hesitancy
  - Frequency
  - Urgency
  - Nocturia
  - Decreased force or interruption of the urine stream
- Neurologic deficits
- Urine leakage when bearing down
- History of urinary tract infection, prostate conditions, spinal injury or tumor, stroke, or surgery involving the bladder, prostate, or pelvic floor

How it's treated

- Pelvic muscle rehabilitation
  - Kegel exercises
  - Pelvic floor electrical stimulation
- Behavior therapies
  - Bladder training
  - Toileting assistance for those who have limited mobility or who require prompting due to forgetfulness
- Medications
  - Oxybutynin to relax sphincter muscles, thus preventing urge incontinence
  - Tolterodine to treat overactive bladder, frequency, urgency, or urge incontinence
  - Estrogen (oral or vaginal form) to improve tone

- Surgery, such as sling procedures and bulking injections, to treat specific anatomical problems
- Management of fluid intake and diet (eliminate caffeine, encourage adequate fiber, reduce fluid intake in the evening)
- Disposable absorbent garments

Varicose veins

- Dilated, tortuous veins, engorged with blood
- Result from improper venous valve function
- Primary
  – Originate in superficial veins
  – Most common
  – Usually bilateral
- Secondary
  – Originate in deep veins
  – Occur in one leg

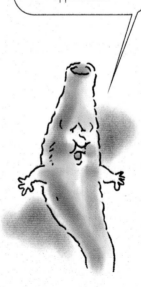

Incompetent venous valves! They're the culprits responsible for my dilated, tortuous appearance.

What causes it

Primary

- Congenital weakness of the valves or venous wall
- Conditions that produce prolonged venous stasis or increased intra-abdominal pressure, such as pregnancy, obesity, constipation, chronic cough, or tight clothes
- Occupations that necessitate standing for an extended period
- Family history

Secondary

- Deep vein thrombosis
- Venous malformation
- Arteriovenous fistulas
- Trauma
- Occlusion

What to look for

- Dilated, tortuous, purplish, ropelike veins, particularly in the calves
- Edema of the calves and ankles
- Leg heaviness or fatigue that worsens in the evening and with warm weather
- Dull aching in the legs after prolonged standing or walking or during menses
- Leg cramps at night
- Itching of the affected area

How it's treated

- Elevation of legs above level of the heart as much as possible
- Antiembolism stockings or elastic bandages to support the veins, improve circulation, and counteract swelling
- Regular exercise to promote venous return
- Dietary modifications to lose weight, avoid alcohol, and avoid constipation with increased fiber
- Analgesics to treat pain and cramping
- Sclerotherapy for small to medium varicosities
- Endovenous laser therapy or radiofrequency ablation to destroy the vein
- Surgical avulsion, stripping, or ligation for severe cases

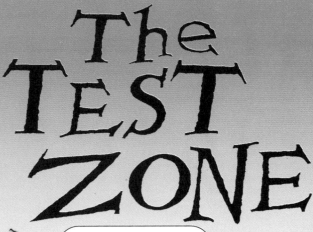

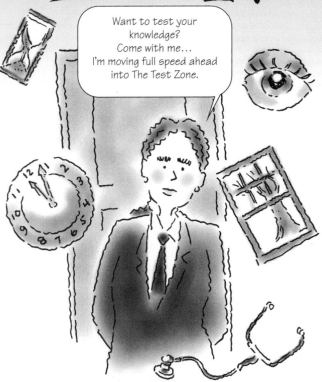

A–B

1. Your patient, diagnosed with adrenal insufficiency, requires lifelong replacement therapy of which substance?
   A. Potassium
   B. Glucose
   C. Corticosteroids
   D. Sodium

2. Angina, syncope, and dyspnea are three classic findings associated with which disorder?
   A. Aortic stenosis
   B. Atrial fibrillation
   C. Pericardial effusion
   D. Digoxin toxicity

3. Your patient is experiencing loss of coordination, disorientation, restlessness, and agitation. These findings are characteristic of which disorder?
   A. Attention deficit hyperactivity disorder
   B. Alzheimer's disease
   C. Generalized anxiety disorder
   D. Alcohol dependence

4. What is generally the first sign of bladder cancer?
   A. Incontinence
   B. Severe pain before voiding
   C. Painless, gross, intermittent hematuria
   D. Superpubic mass

C–G

5. Your patient has been diagnosed with gallstones. What is the treatment of choice for cholelithiasis?
   A. Cholecystectomy
   B. T-tube placement
   C. Dietary management
   D. Pain control

6. Why are beta-adrenergic blockers given to patients with acute coronary syndrome?
   A. To restore vessel patency
   B. To decrease myocardial workload and oxygen demands
   C. To reduce elevated serum cholesterol or triglyceride levels
   D. To inhibit platelet aggregation

7. What dietary modification should be made by patients with diverticular disease?
   A. Avoidance of spicy foods
   B. Low-residual diet
   C. Low-sodium intake
   D. High-fiber intake

8. What is the definition of Type I diabetes?
   A. Pregnancy-related diabetes
   B. Absolute insulin insufficiency
   C. Insulin resistance with varying degrees of insulin secretory defects
   D. Isolated episodes of hyperglycemia

9. Chronic open-angle glaucoma results from overproduction or obstruction of outflow of what substance?
   A. Aqueous humor
   B. Serous fluid
   C. Optic fluid
   D. Tears

H-M

10. Exercise, weight loss, smoking cessation, and reduced intake of sodium, alcohol and fat are lifestyle modifications recommended to treat which condition?

    A. Mitral valve insufficiency

    B. Gout

    C. Hypertension

    D. Lyme disease

11. Immunization is available to prevent which chronic disease?

    A. Hepatitis C

    B. Hepatitis B

    C. Herpes simplex type 2

    D. Irritable bowel disease

12. Hemophilia B is also known as:

    A. classic hemophilia.

    B. clotting factor VIII disease.

    C. thrombocytopenia.

    D. Christmas disease.

13. Asymmetrical lesions with irregular borders, wider than 6 mm, are characteristic of which disorder?

    A. Malignant melanoma

    B. Lupus erythematosus

    C. Macular degeneration

    D. Multiple sclerosis

14. Which arrhythmia occurs most commonly with mitral stenosis?

    A. Atrial fibrillation

    B. Second-degree heart block

    C. Ventricular tachycardia

    D. Sinus bradycardia

N–Z

15. Which finding contributes to the development of renal calculi and infection seen in neurogenic bladder disorders?
    A. Incontinence
    B. Urinary retention
    C. Hypercalcemia
    D. Bladder spasms

16. Osteoclastic and osteoblastic phases occur in which disease?
    A. Paget's disease
    B. Osteoporosis
    C. Osteoarthritis
    D. Ovarian cancer

17. What is the initial treatment of chronic otitis media for a 6-year-old child without hearing loss?
    A. Antibiotic therapy
    B. Ventilation tubes
    C. Watchful waiting for further fluid reabsorption
    D. Anti-inflammatory drug

18. Progressive muscle rigidity, akinesia, and involuntary tremor are manifestations of what neurologic disorder?
    A. Myasthenia gravis
    B. Parkinson's disease
    C. Muscular dystrophy
    D. Peripheral neuralgia

19. A low-protein diet to limit accumulation of end products from protein metabolism is advised in which chronic disorder?
    A. Ulcerative colitis
    B. Renal failure
    C. Stroke
    D. Thalassemia

20. What is the most crucial step in determining treatment of a stroke?
    A. Assessing the extent of paralysis
    B. Obtaining consent from the patient's family
    C. Determining the patient's blood pressure
    D. Differentiating hemorrhagic from ischemic stroke

21. Excess serum iron from frequent blood transfusions is removed from the blood by which process?
    A. Chelation therapy
    B. Phlebotomy
    C. Forcing fluids
    D. Dietary restriction

Answers

A–B

1. C. Adrenal insufficiency requires lifelong corticosteroid replacement therapy.

2. A. Classic findings associated with aortic stenosis include, angina, syncope, and dyspnea.

3. B. Disorientation is an early sign of Alzheimer's disease. As the disease progresses, the patient may also show loss of coordination, restlessness, and agitation.

4. C. The first sign of bladder cancer is commonly painless, gross, intermittent hematuria.

C–G

5. A. Surgery (cholecystectomy) is the treatment of choice for gall-stones.

6. B. Beta-adrenergic blockers are given during acute coronary syndrome to decrease myocardial workload and oxygen demands.

7. D. A high-fiber, high-residual diet is advised for patients with diverticular disease.

8. B. Type I diabetes is defined as absolute insulin insufficiency.

9. A. Overproduction or obstruction of the outflow of aqueous humor from the eye causes the increased intraocular pressure found in glaucoma.

H-M

10. C. Lifestyle modifications recommended in the treatment of hypertension include exercise, weight loss, smoking cessation, and reduced intake of sodium, alcohol and fat.

11. B. Vaccination is available to prevent hepatitis B.

12. D. Hemophilia B is also known as Christmas disease.

13. A. Malignant melanoma lesions are characteristically asymmetrical with irregular borders and more than 6 mm wide.

14. A. The most common arrhythmia that occurs with mitral stenosis is atrial fibrillation.

N–Z

15. B. Urinary retention contributes to the formation of renal calculi and urinary tract infections.

16. A. Abnormal bone resorption (osteoclastic phase) and excessive abnormal bone formation (osteoblastic phase) are the two phases of Paget's disease.

17. C. Initial treatment of chronic otitis media for a child who has developed language skills and is without hearing loss is observation for natural fluid reabsorption.

18. B. Parkinson's disease produces progressive muscle rigidity, akinesia, and involuntary tremor.

19. B. A low-protein diet to limit accumulation of end products of protein metabolism that kidneys can't excrete is recommended in chronic renal failure.

20. D. Differentiating a hemorrhagic stroke from an ischemic stroke is the first crucial step in treatment since the treatment guidelines for one could be life-threatening in the other.

21. A. Chelation therapy is used to bind excess iron for excretion from the body.

Scoring

☆☆☆ If you answered 19 to 21 questions correctly, great job! You're in a dimension all by yourself.

☆☆ If you answered 13 to 18 questions correctly, way to go! You're really in the zone.

☆ If you answered fewer than 13 questions correctly, review the chapters and try again! It won't be long until you see the light.

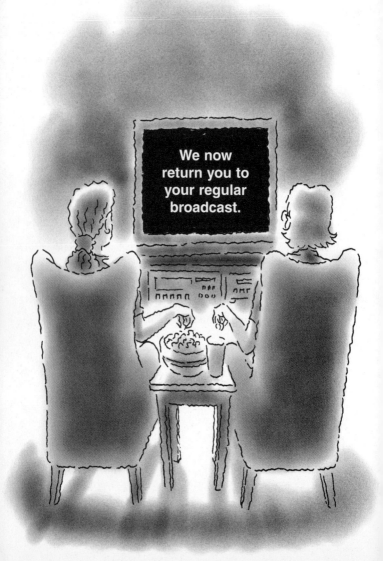

Selected references

Atallah, E., and Cortes, J. "Optimal Initial Therapy for Patients with Newly Diagnosed Chronic Myeloid Leukemia in the Chronic Phase," *Current Opinion in Internal Medicine* 6(3):268-74, June 2007.

Atlas of Pathophysiology, 2nd ed. Philadelphia: Lippincott Williams & Wilkins, 2004.

Coccheri, S. "Approaches to Prevention of Cardiovascular Complications and Events in Diabetes Mellitus,"*Drugs* 67(7):997-1026, 2007.

Diagnostic and Statistical Manual of Mental Disorders, 4th ed. Text revision. Washington, D.C.: American Psychiatric Association, 2000.

Fahey, V. *Vascular Nursing*, 4th ed. Philadelphia: W.B. Saunders Co., 2004.

Hoeger, K.M. "Obesity and Lifestyle Management in Polycystic Ovary Syndrome," *Clinical Obstetrics and Gynecology* 50(1):277-94, March 2007.

Klahr, S. "Progression of Chronic Renal Disease," *Heart Disease* 3(3):205-09, May/June 2001.

Lewis, L. "Discussion and Recommendations: Addressing Barriers in the Management of Cancer Survivors," *AJN* 106 (3 Supp.):91-95, March 2006.

Maher, A. et al. *Orthopaedic Nursing*, 3rd ed. Philadelphia: W.B. Saunders Co., 2002.

Managing Chronic Disorders. Philadelphia: Lippincott Williams & Wilkins, 2006.

Montes, G., and Halterman, J. "Characteristics of School-age Children with Autism," *Journal of Developmental and Behavioral Pediatrics* 27(5):379-85, October 2006.

Pathophysiology Made Incredibly Easy, 3rd ed. Philadelphia: Lippincott Williams & Wilkins, 2006.

Porth, C.M. *Pathophysiology Concepts of Altered Health States*, 7th ed. Philadelphia: Lippincott Williams & Wilkins, 2005.

Nursing 2008 Drug Handbook, 28th ed. Philadelphia: Lippincott Williams & Wilkins, 2008.

RN Expert Guides: Respiratory Care. Philadelphia: Lippincott Williams & Wilkins, 2008.

Specht, J. "9 Myths of Incontinence in Older Adults: Both Clinicians and the Over-65 Set Need to Know More," *AJN* 105(6):58-68, June 2005.

Williams-Gray, C., et al. "Cognitive Deficits and Psychosis in Parkinson's Disease: A Review of Pathophysiology and Therapeutic Options," *CNS Drugs* 20(6):477-505, 2006.

Woods, S.L., et al. *Cardiac Nursing*, 5th ed. Philadelphia: Lippincott Williams & Wilkins, 2005.

Index

i refers to an illustration; t refers to a table.

i refers to an illustration; t refers to a table.

Notes

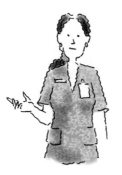

Notes

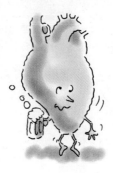

Notes

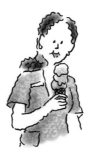

Notes

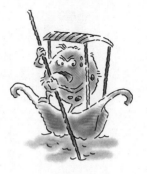

Notes

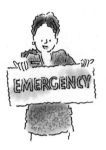

Notes

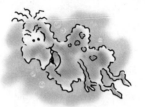